A DEATH IN THE FAMILY

A DEATH IN THE FAMILY

Orphans
of the HIV Epidemic

Edited by

Carol Levine
Executive Director
The Orphan Project

United Hospital Fund of New York

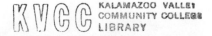

Printed in the United States of America.

Library of Congress Cataloging-in-Publication Data

A Death in the family: orphans of the HIV epidemic/Carol Levine, editor
p. cm.
Includes bibliographical references.
ISBN 1-881277-13-5: $10.00
1. Children of aids patients—Health and hygiene. 2. Children of aids patients—Mental health. 3. Children of aids patients—Services for. 4. Orphans—Health and hygiene. 5. Orphans—Mental health. 6. Orphans—Services for. I. Levine, Carol.

RA644.A25D43 1993
362.1'969792—dc20   93-21517
                                                                              CIP

For information, write, Publications Program, United Hospital Fund, 55 Fifth Avenue, New York, NY 10003.

Cover photograph: © Steve Hart 1993. The photograph is from a work in progress documenting the lives of a family in which both parents have AIDS. Mr. Hart's contribution to *A Death in the Family* was facilitated by Visual AIDS, a diverse group of artists and art workers concerned about AIDS and dedicated to the explication and exposition of the ever-increasing body of art about AIDS.

Contents

Foreword

IN THE PAST DECADE, AIDS has altered the shape of our communities, with families as well as individuals being lost to the disease. Attempting to respond, governments allocate more funds for AIDS each year but find themselves looking up the side of a bigger mountain in terms of what is needed.

Sometimes we are called upon to do something entirely above and beyond incremental change. Those left orphaned by the AIDS epidemic present some of the most difficult needs of all and expose the inadequacies of our current service systems to meet the needs of youth in general. The professionals who provide our children with health, educational, and social services, in addition to their own strength and creativity, must have resources available to fund their efforts. Most importantly, the families who are affected by AIDS must get the support they need to continue with their lives.

The plight of the children who survive a parent's death from AIDS, of the parents who must leave their children to the care of others, and of the new guardians themselves is voiced clearly and compellingly through the work of The Orphan Project. Founded in 1991 by Carol Levine, who received a 1993 MacArthur Fellowship in recognition of her pathfinding work, the group conducts research, advocates for policy and programs, and generally sounds the alarm on this crisis.

In October 1992, The Orphan Project and the United Hospital Fund brought together more than 400 health care and social service providers and advocates for the nation's first conference on this deepening legacy of AIDS. This book is one product of that meeting. By bringing the words of the conference participants to others who work with youth and families, to policymakers, and to the public, we hope to stimulate further collaboration around this pressing social issue.

"What affects a few of us often will have some eventual impact upon the rest of us." These words, from *AIDS Public Policy Dimensions*, published by the Fund seven years ago, are fulfilled in persuasive detail throughout the following pages. In the second decade of the AIDS catastrophe, we will continue to seek ways to improve services for all those affected by the disease and to develop policies that recognize our common stake in accessible and humane care.

JAMES R. TALLON, JR.
President
United Hospital Fund of New York

Preface

THIS BOOK BEGAN in the spring of 1992 as an idea for a small conference. At that time—a year after its inception—The Orphan Project had identified several key issues to be considered in developing programs and policies for private and public agencies working with families in which there are youngsters whose parents are living with HIV/AIDS or who have already died of the disease. The Project had also found that a number of people in New York City had a wealth of experience and insight into these problems. Why not, we thought, bring some of this experience to a larger group? We knew we would also learn much from the audience.

When approached with this idea for a modest conference, the United Hospital Fund staff reacted enthusiastically and efficiently. The conference was held on October 29, 1992. The expected audience of 100 participants grew to over 400, with many more turned away for lack of space.

Because of the overwhelming response to the conference itself and the participants' repeated requests for more information, we decided to produce a small book based on the conference presentations. Once again the subject and its urgency led to an expansion of the original goals. While derived in large part from the conference, this volume goes far beyond it.

Both the conference and the book owe their existence to many people's dedication and excellent work. At the United Hospital Fund, David Gould, Sally Rogers, Jo Ann Silverstein, Deborah Halper, Brenda Lamb, and Carla Fine were instrumental in planning, publicizing, and coordinating the conference. At The Orphan Project, Gary Stein, Ken Chu, and Ben Munisteri provided valuable assistance. Because they are not specifically represented in the book, we especially want to note the following people who participated at the conference as workshop facilitators: Ruth Bezares, founder and director of Mothers of Children with AIDS (MOCA); Sylvia Muniz, supervisor of HIV projects at The Door; Diane Pincus Strom, associate director of social work, Bronx-Lebanon Hospital Center; Katie O'Neill, HIV/AIDS project director, Legal Action Center; Diane LaGamma, Community Law Offices of the Legal Aid Society; and Elizabeth Cox Avedon, cofounder of the Mayer-Avedon Women's Support Groups.

Moving from the spoken to the written word required the additional efforts of many people. At the United Hospital Fund, Avery Hudson and Liza Buffaloe managed the editing and production processes, with a special contribution by Karyn Feiden. At The Orphan Project, Ken Chu provided both administrative assistance and computer expertise in creating the figures in Chapter 1. Gary Stein read and commented on several portions of the manuscript. Ben Munisteri undertook his assignment as assistant to the editor with extraordinary skill and perseverance. He edited manuscripts; telephoned, faxed, and cajoled authors; and managed to keep the many parts of this volume on track. He developed the survey on which the Resource Guide is based and prepared the Resource Guide itself, as well as the Bibliography.

All the authors have our sincere thanks for their contributions. A special acknowledgment, however, goes to the authors who have shared their lives and their most private concerns with us and the readers of this book. This book is immeasurably richer for their candor and courage.

CAROL LEVINE

Introduction

Carol Levine

*Carol Levine is the executive director of
The Orphan Project, New York City.*

IN REVIEWING THE 15 leading causes of death in the United States for 1989, the Centers for Disease Control and Prevention (CDC) noted the sharp increase—33 percent from the previous year—in deaths related to HIV infection. In a departure from its typically laconic scientific prose, the CDC commented: "The recognition of a disease and its emergence as a leading cause of death within the same decade is without precedent."[1]

Nearly three quarters of HIV-related adult deaths occurred among men and women aged 25 to 44—the prime reproductive years. Because of the epidemic's early and devastating spread among gay men in the United States, the majority of AIDS cases have been reported among men. But AIDS among women—present since the beginning—is moving forward rapidly. Women made up 9 percent of the first 100,000 cases of AIDS, but 12 percent of the second 100,000.[2] That trend is expected to continue. By 1989, AIDS had become the sixth leading cause of death nationwide among women 25 to 44 years of age, and the second leading cause of death of men in this age group. The impact of HIV on mortality has been particularly grave in New York City.[3]

These statistics represent not only the tragic loss of individual lives; they warn of a crisis in family and societal responsibility. Most of these dying women and many of the men leave children. Some of the surviving children were infected with HIV through maternal-fetal transmission, but the vast majority are not infected with the virus. They range from infants to older adolescents and young adults. Like their parents, they come primarily from poor communities of color. When their parents die, some of these children need new sources of shelter, food, and medical care, and all of them need emotional support and guidance.

If the rapid emergence of HIV/AIDS as a lethal disease is without precedent, it also seems plausible that the rapid emergence of this group of particularly vulnerable parentless children is also without precedent, at least in our country in our century. Tuberculosis also took a heavy toll among young adults in the 19th and early 20th centuries, but that disease is centuries old. Only the great influenza pandemic of 1918, which swept the world and took young and old in its wake, offers a partial analogy from diseases of the 20th century.

This book, like the conference that was its genesis, is devoted to this phenomenon. Both derive from the work of The Orphan Project, an organization devoted to study, analysis, and advocacy for policies and programs that meet the needs of children surviving a parent's death from HIV/AIDS. The project does not provide direct services; it encourages public understanding, support, and allocation of the resources necessary to create and implement direct services in the community. The project is administered by the Fund for the City of New York and is supported by foundation grants.* As important as the specific activities is the opportunity to bring together people who are working more or less independently and to help them form coalitions and networks.

Although, as Chapter 1 demonstrates, the problem of surviving youth is already staggering, we are only at the beginning of this phenomenon. We do not know its duration, its sweep, or many of its consequences. We do know that a great many children and families have already suffered many losses and that the future looks bleak. But this book is also a testimony to the many people who have exhibited strength, resiliency, courage, and resourcefulness in the face of enormous adversity.

This volume focuses on surviving children and adolescents—their needs and those of their families and new guardians. In doing so, we do not intend to neglect the others in their families, particularly their ill

---

*The Altman Foundation, the American Foundation for AIDS Research, the Conanima Foundation, the Fund for the City of New York, the Ittleson Foundation, the Joyce Mertz-Gilmore Foundation, the New York City AIDS Fund, the New York Life Foundation, the Norman and Rosita Winston Foundation, the Prudential Foundation, the Robert Wood Johnson Foundation, the Rockefeller Brothers Fund, and the United Hospital Fund.

parents. One of the most important things we can do for children in this epidemic is to keep their parents well as long as possible, so that together they can build a memory bank of good times and share the bad times. Because they are most often the primary caregivers, mothers especially need the best possible medical care, social services, and financial and legal assistance so that they can be a positive force in their children's lives and can plan for the ultimate future.

Nor should we forget the fathers, even though much of this book focuses on mothers. Fathers also play a special role in children's lives, and it is only because for most children their mothers are the primary caregivers that we concentrate on them.

Finally, we should remember that children from families with HIV/AIDS are not the only children in our city who need our care and attention. They are both like and different from other children who face a family or community crisis. What sets these children apart and generates our special concern for them is a particular combination of vulnerabilities. All children who lose a parent suffer a permanent and profound loss. As psychiatrist Paul Buttenweiser puts it:

> Children who have lost a parent often speak of a tremendous chasm opening up, a sense of an unbridgeable divide separating events that happened before from all that came after. They attempt, often unconsciously, to make contact with the "other side," trying to overcome the sense of unauthenticity that shrouds their lives. They do this in various ways, most importantly in the relationships and families they establish for themselves, and in their creative efforts—although loss can be a spur as well as a barrier to both those endeavors.[4]

Children whose parents die of HIV/AIDS undergo a particularly wounding experience that encompasses stigma, secrecy, and denial as they witness their parents' physical and often mental deterioration. When a parent's death is accompanied by stigma and isolation, and is followed by instability and insecurity, the potential for trouble, both immediately and in the future, is magnified.

All children whose families are torn apart by violence, homelessness, or other social ills are profoundly affected by these crises. But those children whose families endure AIDS as well as these other deprivations are doubly affected. It is our hope that policies and programs aimed at the children who survive parents with AIDS will highlight the needs of all our children.

This book describes the problem from many different perspectives, including epidemiology, law, mental health, program development, advocacy, and personal experience. Part I presents results of research on the numbers of youth who will survive the death of their mothers from HIV/AIDS in New York City and the findings of a pioneering study of the mental health needs of well adolescents in families with AIDS. Part II contains several personal experiences of family members affected by HIV/AIDS. Part III treats several important issues that each family must address: questions of bereavement and the various ways in which children express their grief; questions of confidentiality and disclosure of HIV-related information in a societal context of stigma and avoidance; and legal questions of planning for the future custody and care of the children. Part IV offers several models of innovative programs that are addressing different aspects of the needs of families and youngsters. A set of recommendations for service, research, education, and training follows in Part V. Finally, a resource guide directs readers to services currently available in New York City and a selected bibliography provides readings for adults and children.

This book focuses on the concrete needs of families living with disease and the threat of death. Sometimes, however, the most perceptive expressions of reality come not from facts or policies but from the life of the imagination, from fiction. Here, then, is a passage from the novel that gave the conference and this book their title—James Agee's *A Death in the Family*, published in 1955.

Set in Knoxville, Tennessee, in 1915, the novel depicts the impact on the family when a young father of two children dies in an automobile accident. After learning of his father's death the next morning, the boy, Rufus, rises from the breakfast table:

> When breakfast was over he wandered listlessly into the sitting room and looked all around, but he did not see any place where he would like to sit down. He felt deeply idle and at the same time gravely exhilarated, as if this were the morning of his birthday, except that this day seemed even more particularly his own day. There was nothing in the way it looked which was not ordinary, but it was filled with a noiseless and invisible kind of energy. He could see his mother's face while she told them about it and hear her voice, over and over, and silently, over and over, while he looked around the sitting room and through the window into the street, words repeated themselves. He's dead. He died last night while I was asleep and now it was already morning. He has already been dead since way last night and I didn't even know un-

til I woke up. He has been dead all night while I was asleep and he will stay right on being dead all afternoon and all night and all tomorrow while I am asleep again and wake up again and go to sleep again and he can't come back home again ever any more but I will see him once more before he is taken away. Dead now. He died last night while I was asleep and now it is already morning.[5]

In this lyrical passage Agee captures a child's confrontation with the finality of death. Each of us, in our own ways, can help make that confrontation a source of understanding and growth. Together we can make a difference in creating the strong policy and programmatic base necessary to meet this challenge.

Notes

1. Centers for Disease Control. "Mortality Patterns—United States, 1989," *Morbidity and Mortality Weekly Report* 41 (1992):121.
2. Centers for Disease Control. "The second 100,000 Cases of Acquired Immunodeficiency Syndrome, " *Morbidity and Mortality Weekly Report* 41 (1992):28-29.
3. Selik, R.M.; Chu, S.Y.; Buehler, J.W. "HIV Infection as Leading Cause of Death Among Young Adults in US Cities and States," *Journal of the American Medical Association* 269 (1993):2991-2994.
4. Buttenweiser, P. *New York Times Book Review*. October 25, 1992, p. 22.
5. Agee, J. *A Death in the Family* (New York: Putnam, 1955). From *A Death in the Family* by James Agee, copyright © 1957 by The James Agee Trust, copyright © renewed 1985 by Mia Agee. Reprinted by permission of Grosset & Dunlap, Inc.

I

THE DIMENSIONS OF
THE PROBLEM

1

The Youngest Survivors: Estimates of the Number of Motherless Youth Orphaned by AIDS in New York City

David Michaels, Carol Levine

David Michaels, Ph.D., M.P.H., is associate professor of epidemiology in the Department of Community Health and Social Medicine at the City University of New York Medical School/Sophie Davis School of Biomedical Education, New York City.

Carol Levine is the executive director of The Orphan Project, New York City.

FROM THE FIRST FIVE cases of a mysterious syndrome reported to the U.S. Centers for Disease Control and Prevention (CDC) in 1981 to the millions of cases of HIV infection estimated by the World Health Organization (WHO) today, epidemiologists have tried to quantify almost all aspects of the rising tide of the AIDS epidemic.

Since the beginning of the epidemic, New York City has led the nation in many of these statistics. Of the national total of 315,390 reported cases of AIDS (through June 30, 1993), New York City has accounted for nearly 52,000, or about 16 percent.[1,2] According to the New York City Department of Health, in 1990 AIDS was the third leading cause of death for men of all ages and the leading cause of death for men from the ages of 25 through 34 (33.8 percent) and from 35 through 44 (39.3 percent). AIDS was the leading cause of death for women aged 25 through 44 (30.2 percent), and the leading cause of death of African-American women aged 15 through 44.[3]

Even though, as these statistics demonstrate, the epidemic has hit hard at women and men in their prime reproductive years, only in the past few years has a basic question been raised: How many children are surviving the death of a parent of an HIV/AIDS-related cause? To date, there have been no solid answers to this fundamental question.

People living and working in the hardest hit communities have known many families with surviving children, but there has been no epidemiologic model to estimate their actual number. The Orphan Project took as one of its first tasks the development of such a model for New York City and the United States.

An Invisible Population

The various categories of children and adolescents who are infected with or affected by HIV can be represented schematically in the form of an iceberg (Exhibit 1-1). The tip of the iceberg represents the approximately 5,000 pediatric AIDS cases in the United States reported to the CDC (including the small number of reported adolescent cases). Understandably, pediatric AIDS has received the most public and professional attention, since these very sick children and their families have urgent medical and social service needs. Just below the tip of the iceberg, and only partially visible above the water line, are known cases of HIV-infected children and adolescents. That there are many more HIV-infected newborns than known pediatric AIDS cases (more than three times as many in 1989,[4] for example) means that a large portion of this section of the iceberg is still hidden.

The next largest portion of the iceberg represents the uninfected siblings of the group with AIDS or HIV infection. These may be older brothers and sisters, born before their mother contracted HIV, or younger children who escaped maternal-fetal transmission. (Current rates of maternal-fetal transmission in the New York City area are about 30 percent—lower than those in Africa but considerably higher than those in Europe, for still unexplained reasons.[5]) By far the largest and most hidden portion of the iceberg is the one represented by diagonally shaded lines in the illustration. This portion includes uninfected children and adolescents whose parent or parents, another adult relative, or a person who although unrelated by birth or marriage has come to be considered family either has died of AIDS or is living with AIDS or serious HIV disease. To carry the image one step further, the iceberg itself is situated in a stormy sea of violence, homelessness, drug abuse, poverty, discrimination, and societal neglect.

Exhibit 1-1
Children and Adolescents Affected by HIV/AIDS

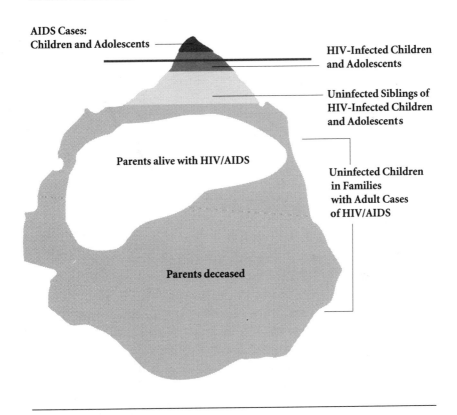

AIDS Cases:
Children and Adolescents

HIV-Infected Children
and Adolescents

Uninfected Siblings of
HIV-Infected Children
and Adolescents

Parents alive with HIV/AIDS

Uninfected Children
in Families
with Adult Cases
of HIV/AIDS

Parents deceased

Defining Orphans

Although in recent years the term "orphan" has been used most commonly to describe a child who has lost both parents, throughout Western history the term has been used to define a child who has lost either one or both parents.

A definition that focuses on motherless youth was chosen because, for the vast majority of youth whose caregiving parent dies of HIV/AIDS, that parent is the mother. There are, of course, families in which an uninfected father is willing and able to serve as primary caregiver when the mother dies of AIDS. These situations appear to be rare, however. There are also families in which the death of the father from AIDS, even when the mother is uninfected, is a traumatic event that results in breakup of the family. Although both scenarios are important in developing programs to meet the range of individual needs, they do not affect the broad epidemiological picture.

The definition also conforms to the realities of epidemiological analysis, because there are few data on the offspring of men dying of HIV disease. For these reasons, this definition is used by the CDC,[6] WHO, and the United Nations Children's Fund (UNICEF).[7] If data on fathers were available, it would be possible to estimate the number of children who will lose their fathers to the epidemic, which would dramatically increase the number of children reported here. However, there are no statistics available for men that are the equivalent of fertility rates among women. Because no one has calculated the general rate at which men father children, it is impossible to estimate how many children will be left fatherless because of HIV/AIDS. Even so, a series of studies of selected populations of men (in drug treatment centers, for example) would provide data to illuminate this important question.

Orphans of the Epidemic in New York City

Through the end of 1992, approximately 4,800 children and 4,500 adolescents are estimated to have been orphaned by HIV/AIDS in New York City (Exhibit 1-2). As projections move into more distant time, they inevitably become less precise. Unless the course of the epidemic changes dramatically, however, by the year 2000 the cumulative number will include 15,000 who were orphaned as children and another 15,000 orphaned as adolescents.

The range of ages of these orphans is particularly notable. In addition to young children, a large number of adolescents are being, or will be, orphaned. Their needs are very different from those of infants or children.

In addition to these sizable groups, 25,000 young adults (those 18 years and older) will lose their mothers to the disease. Although the needs of this group may at first seem less emotionally compelling than those of their younger brothers and sisters, they are nonetheless significant. Particularly if they assume responsibility for the care of younger siblings, these young adults will also face serious psychosocial, financial, and legal problems.

According to current estimates, more than 80 percent of the youth orphaned by HIV/AIDS in New York City are offspring of women of color (Exhibit 1-3). The categories ("white," "Hispanic," "black") are designated by the CDC; they reflect the data that are made available to researchers. Not surprisingly, the highest concentrations of these orphans are in

Exhibit 1-2
**Motherless Youth Orphaned by HIV/AIDS
Cumulative by Age Category, New York City
1982–2000**

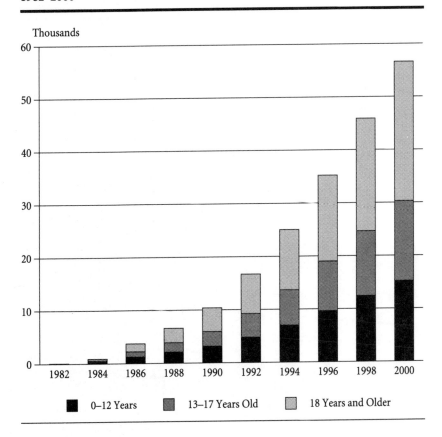

Brooklyn, the Bronx, and Manhattan, where most of the HIV-infected women reside (Exhibit 1-4).

Building the Model

Where did these numbers come from? The starting point was the number of reported and projected AIDS deaths among adult women younger than 50 years old. These numbers were then adjusted for the documented undercount of HIV-related mortality among women.[8] Then these numbers were applied to age, race/ethnicity, and calendar-specific cumulative fertility rates, permitting an estimation of the number of children these women might have borne, and when. The results were then further ad-

Exhibit 1-3

**Motherless Children and Adolescents Orphaned by HIV/AIDS
Cumulative by Race/Ethnicity, New York City
1982–2000**

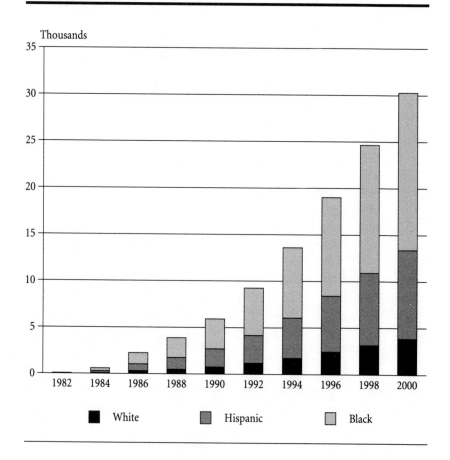

justed for decreased fertility associated with late-stage HIV disease, infant mortality, and pediatric AIDS mortality.*

Whatever assumptions go into the model, the overall picture remains basically the same. Exhibit 1-5 shows three estimates of children and adolescents left motherless by HIV/AIDS, based on a range of values for the

---

* The methods used to construct this model are explained in greater detail in David Michaels and Carol Levine, "Estimates of the Number of Motherless Youth Orphaned by AIDS in the United States," *Journal of the American Medical Association* 268 (December 23/30, 1992):3456-3461.

Exhibit 1-4
Estimated Distribution of Motherless Children and Adolescents Orphaned by HIV/AIDS, by New York City Borough

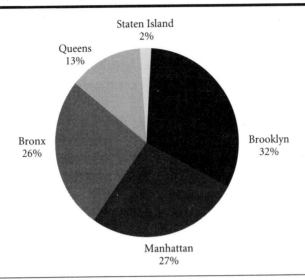

proportions of HIV-related deaths that are identified on death certificates, the pediatric AIDS and overall infant mortality rates, the number of projected AIDS deaths among women in the future, and other parameters used in the model. In the low end of the range, 29,000 children and adolescents will be orphaned by the year 2000; the high estimate is more than 34,000. The model is based on fairly conservative assumptions (for example, the middle estimate follows current predictions, probably over-optimistic, that the annual number of AIDS deaths will stop increasing after 1995); therefore, the estimates should not be considered as overstatements of the problem.

The View from the Nation
The problem in New York is part of a larger, national problem. Consider two projections of the number of youth orphaned by HIV/AIDS nationally. Using the same model described for New York City, we estimate that, unless the course of the epidemic changes dramatically, by the year 2000 the overall number of motherless children and adolescents in the United States will exceed 80,000 (range 72,000 to 125,000).

HIV/AIDS has come to rival or surpass other important causes of death in taking the lives of mothers of young children nationally. Among women

Exhibit 1-5
Motherless Children and Adolescents Orphaned by HIV/AIDS
Cumulative, New York City
1981–2000

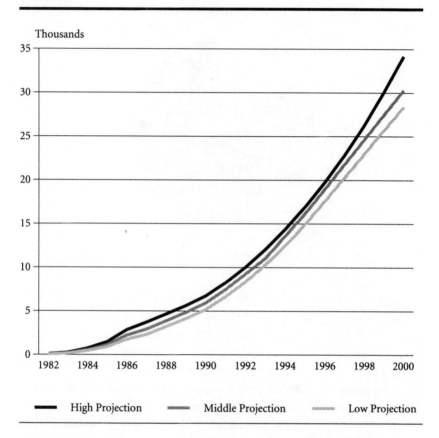

Thousands

High Projection   Middle Projection   Low Projection

under the age of 50, cancer is the cause of death of mothers of approximately 4,200 children and 8,700 adolescents annually. Motor vehicle accidents are responsible for the deaths of mothers of an additional 3,200 children and 1,900 adolescents. In contrast, the numbers of children and adolescents annually left motherless by HIV are predicted to reach 3,900 and 3,400, respectively, by 1993.

Using a different model, the CDC arrived at a similar estimate, predicting that between 93,000 and 112,000 uninfected children will be born to mothers who die of HIV/AIDS between 1992 and the year 2000. Additionally, these women will give birth to between 32,000 and 38,000 children infected with HIV during the decade.[6]

Five years ago, more than half of the children orphaned by HIV/AIDS in the nation lived in New York City. By 1993, less than one in three will live there. Unfortunately, this proportion is decreasing not because the epidemic is subsiding in New York, but because the rate of AIDS deaths among women is rising even more rapidly elsewhere.

Other cities with large numbers of reported AIDS cases among women are Newark, Miami, San Juan, Los Angeles, and Washington, DC. However, children affected by the epidemic will not be limited to these metropolitan areas. As the epidemic becomes more deeply entrenched in inner cities, it is also spreading to other cities and even to rural areas throughout the country. And wherever there are women with AIDS, there will be motherless youth.

As the HIV epidemic unfolds, some changes may occur in the age distribution. For example, the women represented in mortality statistics so far have been mainly in their thirties and forties. As younger women become infected with HIV and develop AIDS, the proportion of younger children who are orphaned may be expected to increase.

The Challenge for the Future

These findings warn of a serious challenge to cities and communities already staggering under the weight of faltering economies, violence, homelessness, inadequate medical care, poor education, drug abuse, and a host of other long-standing social problems. Yet the needs of these youngsters cannot be ignored. To do so would not only show a lack of compassion for the most vulnerable members of society; it would also invite a social catastrophe of the greatest magnitude. More study is needed on the impact of the HIV epidemic on families, but there is already ample evidence to warrant immediate action, with appropriate evaluation and follow-up. Children and adolescents orphaned by HIV/AIDS cannot wait for the normally slow policy process to address their complex and individualized needs. While some bereaved children and adolescents are already in foster care, and others have been taken in by relatives, most face futures beset by uncertainty and instability, separation from siblings, and unrecognized and unaddressed grief.

Those who develop, interpret, and implement guidelines and programs of custody decisions, foster care, adoption, education, juvenile justice, health care, and institutionalization face a daunting challenge. They must find strength, flexibility, and creativity to address these urgent needs.

Notes

1. Centers for Disease Control and Prevention. *HIV/AIDS Surveillance Report.* Second Quarter Edition, July 1993.

2. New York City Department of Health, Office of AIDS Surveillance. *AIDS Surveillance Update.* Second Quarter 1993.

3. New York City Department of Health. *Summary of Vital Statistics.* 1989.

4. Oxtoby, M.J. "Perinatally Acquired HIV Infection." In Pizzo, P.A.; Wilfert, C.M., eds. *Pediatric AIDS* (Baltimore: Williams & Wilkins, 1991), 9-10.

5. Boylan, L.; Stein, Z.A. "The Epidemiology of HIV Infection in Children and Their Mothers—Vertical Transmission," *Epidemiologic Reviews* 13 (1991):143-177.

6. Caldwell, M.B.; Fleming, P.L.; Oxtoby, M.J. "Estimated Number of AIDS Orphans in the United States," *Pediatrics* 90 (1992):482.

7. United Nations Children's Fund. *Report on a Meeting about AIDS and Orphans in Africa, Florence 14/15 June 1991* (New York: United Nations Children's Fund, 1991), 5-6.

8. Buehler, J.W.; Hanson, D.L.; Chu, S.Y. "The Reporting of HIV/AIDS Deaths in Women," *American Journal of Public Health* 82 (1992):1500-1505.

2

Adolescents in Families with AIDS: Growing Up with Loss

Barbara Draimin

Barbara Draimin, DSW, is the director of planning at the Division of AIDS Services, New York City Human Resources Administration.

THE NUMBER OF ADOLESCENTS living in families with AIDS has risen exponentially over the past five years. In June 1993, the New York City Human Resources Administration's (HRA) Division of AIDS Services (DAS), which provides comprehensive social services for Medicaid-eligible people with AIDS, served 13,629 clients, including 2,492 families. More than 850 of these families had at least one adolescent in the household. Since the beginning of the epidemic, DAS has managed over 42,000 cases, including 6,000 families. The number of families served by DAS, many of them including adolescents, is expected to increase by 33 percent in 1994. Ninety-one percent of the families served by DAS are of Latin or African descent, and the majority of households are headed by single women who are current or former substance users.

In 1991, as part of an ongoing effort to remain informed about client needs and to design innovative programs to address those needs, DAS conducted a study of the mental health needs of well adolescents aged 10 through 19 in 40 families with AIDS.*

---

*Barbara Draimin, Jan Hudis, and José Segura, *The Mental Health Needs of Well Adolescents in Families with AIDS* (New York: Human Resources Administration, 1992). Single copies of the report are available from Barbara Draimin, Division of AIDS Services, Human Resources Administration, 241 Church Street, New York, NY 10013.

Study Findings

The research team (Barbara Draimin, Jan Hudis, and José Segura) conducted three-hour in-home interviews with 40 families. In 20 of these families the parent was living with AIDS, and both the parent and the adolescent were interviewed. In 20 additional families, the parent had died of AIDS, and the new guardian and the adolescent were interviewed. Standardized tests measuring the teenager's self-esteem, anxiety, and depression were also given.

On average, the adolescents in the study had experienced four major losses (through death, divorce, or incarceration of a significant other, for example) in the previous two years. More than 80 percent had experienced at least one such loss. Thirty-four percent of the adolescents interviewed were acting out at home, 73 percent had problems in school, and 58 percent had experienced a decline in school grades associated with their parent's illness. Twenty-five percent of the adolescent boys had recent experience with law enforcement; three had been jailed.

These adolescents had very weak social support networks. Almost 40 percent had no best friend. Thirty-nine percent did not know the HIV status of their living or deceased parent.* Of the 61 percent of the adolescents who knew their parent's diagnosis, none had shared that information with their best friend. These findings demonstrate the isolation of these youth and the stigma surrounding AIDS in the family. On the more positive side, 43 percent of the youth had obtained some form of counseling and 76 percent of these had found the counseling satisfactory.

The two groups of adolescents—those whose parent was alive and those whose parent had died—did not differ significantly from each other or from national norms on measures of self-esteem, depression, and anxiety. Using a standard test of parental reporting, however, we found that 25 percent of the adolescents were exhibiting depressive symptoms severe enough to be considered appropriate for clinical evaluation. These data indicate that although adolescents in families with AIDS are distressed, the majority do not exhibit psychopathology.

---

*DAS clients were invited to participate by means of a letter describing the study, in general terms, as a study of clients' feelings about illness. The team carefully avoided using the terms "AIDS" and "HIV" until the study participant had used them. This was done to protect confidentiality among family members, and out of respect for each family's decision on how to handle disclosure of the parent's HIV status to the children.

When teenagers were asked to list their wishes and dreams, the two most common responses were to have a mother and father and to live in a country without drugs (Exhibit 2-1).

The teens were asked, on anonymous written questionnaires, about their own sex and drug behavior. Their responses showed that they understood the dangers of drugs and AIDS: little drug use was reported. However, they had not heeded the message about the risks of sexual behavior. Boys and girls alike reported having unprotected sex. When an adolescent can be a daily witness to the suffering of a parent with AIDS and still continue to have unprotected sex, there is much educational work to be done.

Interviews with parents and new guardians documented families' difficulties with disclosure and custody planning. In 53 percent of the families where the parent with AIDS was alive there was no viable custody plan for the adolescents. In these families, it was not unusual for a relative to agree

Exhibit 2-1
Wishes and Dreams

If you could have any three wishes in the world, what would you wish for?

Youth who have lost a parent to AIDS answered

- To have my mother back, have fun, and be grown up.

- To have my mother alive, to have a mother and father, and to live in a world where there were no drugs, lying, or stealing.

- To not be left back in school, to go to camp, and to have a lot of money.

- To be rich, for everyone to be immortal, and to have an infinite number of wishes.

Youth who are living with a parent with AIDS answered

- To cure my mother, to do well in school, and for the world to be good.

- To have 100 more wishes, for my mother and family to be in perfect health, and for friends and family to live across the street.

- For my father to be alive, for my mother to feel better, and for us to live in a bigger house.

- To have a drug-free country, to live where no one would ever die, and to live with my Aunt Susan.

to be the guardian for younger children while refusing responsibility for an adolescent—particularly if the adolescent had behavioral problems. In some families, older adolescents fought for guardianship of their young siblings in order to keep all the children together.

Despite their hardships, the families mustered extraordinary reserves of strength and power. Single mothers coping with their own terminal illness demonstrated enormous care and compassion for their children, many of whom had complex needs. Family members, particularly the mothers and sisters of the women with AIDS, were the glue holding these families together. With AIDS in some communities taking the lives of an entire generation of young parents, it was not unusual to interview a grandmother or an aunt caring for the children of more than one daughter or sister. Amid enormous loss, these families moved forward with a strong spirit. The cases of Margaret and Annie (not their real names) illustrate how two families have struggled with disclosure and custody planning.

Margaret
Margaret lives with her family in Brooklyn (Exhibit 2-2). She is originally from Puerto Rico and still has some family there. Margaret was diagnosed with AIDS and became a DAS client in the summer of 1990, when she was hospitalized for two months with pneumonia. Margaret and her physicians attribute much of her physical fragility to extreme stress associated with managing a household of seven, including four teenagers (two with serious behavioral problems) and an infant grandson, all in a small apartment that affords little privacy.

Two of the teenagers (Ralph, 18, and George, 15) are Margaret's nephews, who have been living with Margaret since 1988, when the Child Welfare Administration (CWA) removed them from their mother's household. Currently they have no contact with their mother, a crack addict who had been reported to CWA for neglect and abuse.

Each of Margaret's children has a different father, none of whom is currently involved to any significant extent with the family. Margaret separated three years ago from her husband of seven years, a cocaine addict who is generally manipulative and unreliable. Margaret's most recent partner is not available to care for her or the children. Other family members are only marginally involved; none can provide ongoing support or can be depended on to provide assistance in case of emergency.

Custody arrangements have been made for Margaret's two minor children (Maria, 15, and Manuel, 8), with Margaret's second sister as the future

Exhibit 2-2
The Case of Margaret

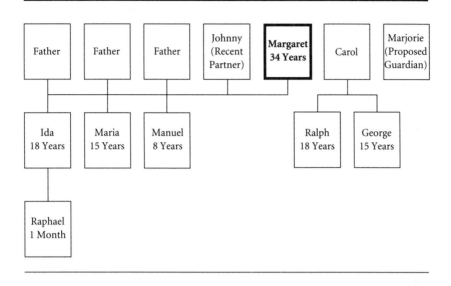

guardian. However, these arrangements are now in question owing to the teenage daughter's defiance at home and at school and her sometimes violent aggressiveness toward her peers. Margaret considers Maria to be her biggest problem at present, and focuses most of her attention in her own counseling sessions on her growing despair about Maria's future and on their inability to communicate. Margaret is also concerned about both of her daughters' unprotected sexual activity with multiple partners.

Manuel is very bright, and started school in an accelerated program for gifted children. Since Margaret's diagnosis and illness, however, his school performance has declined, and now Margaret describes him as easily distracted and unable to concentrate.

Margaret believes that her disclosure of her HIV status to the children, which she made on the advice of her hospital counselor, has had many negative consequences. Her children are now in denial, and unwilling to address Margaret's death with Margaret or anyone else. Margaret believes Maria has not spoken to anyone about her mother's illness, not even to her two best friends. The team's interview with Maria confirmed that she was hiding this information to protect herself and her mother.

As a single parent, Margaret is acutely aware of her children's dependence on her for love, support, care, and discipline. Her children's vulnerability weighs heavily upon Margaret as she thinks about how her illness has disrupted their lives.

Annie

Annie died of AIDS in December 1990 (Exhibit 2-3). Her three children live with their maternal grandmother, Rosie. The youngest, Maddy, is five years old, infected with HIV, and symptomatic. She does not know what her illness is. Her health is fairly good right now, and she is attending school regularly. A home attendant helps with Maddy's care when she returns from school, and she receives visiting nurse services every three weeks.

Rosie and her family are from Haiti, and they maintain close ties with family and friends there. Rosie is 71 years old and speaks and understands very little English. Annie's sister, Marie, is very involved with the family and very close to Rosie. Marie is a nurse; she assists Rosie in negotiating the social service system, relieves her of child care responsibilities when possible, and is generally available for companionship and support.

Exhibit 2-3
The Case of Annie

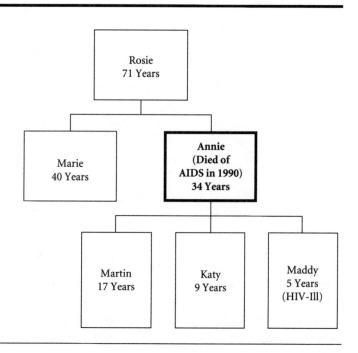

To date, there has been no open acknowledgment among the children that Annie had AIDS or that Maddy is HIV-ill. Rosie and Marie need assistance in deciding whether to talk with the two older children living in the house (Martin, 17 years; Katy, 9 years) about the cause of their mother's death and Maddy's HIV infection. Rosie and Marie believe that Martin knows that his mother had AIDS, even though no one has told him directly. They are uncertain about whether Katy knows.

The entire family is in the early stages of grieving for Annie. Four months after Annie's death, Rosie says she still sees her wasted away in her bed. The sickroom is unused and still contains medical equipment from Annie's last months at home. They all are having a very hard time coping with their feelings, and are reluctant to talk.

Martin has told no one about his mother's death. Martin's football coach, to whom he is very close, found out about Annie's death several months later—and then only through talking with Marie about Martin's declining school performance. Martin wants to go to college to become either an architect or a graphic artist, but he has not been doing as well as usual at school and lately has been getting involved in fights.

Program Implications

Families with AIDS function along a continuum from desperation to hopefulness and from helplessness to self-sufficiency. Although many of the families interviewed by the team demonstrated remarkable reserves of strength and an unusual ability to rally in the face of profound difficulties, their coping skills were inevitably strained by the demands of progressive illness. To help these families confront their losses and build a future, the following strategies should be implemented immediately.

Bereavement Counseling

The families in the study had a great deal to say to someone who was ready to listen. Despite this responsiveness to interviewers, however, most of the family members had virtually no one with whom they discussed their losses. As already noted, not a single teenager had told a best friend that a family member had AIDS. In one case, fear of losing vital church support caused a man with AIDS and his wife to decide against disclosing his HIV status to their fellow parishioners—even though they were active members of a church group that made regular visits to hospitalized AIDS patients.

Short-term in-home counseling for both adults and youth in families with AIDS may help to stabilize their situations. Many families are open to the idea of counseling; however, multiple barriers can exist, including fear of the mental health system, lack of transportation, ethnic and language differences, and long waiting lists at community mental health centers.

Most families do better with home visits, which accommodate their need for privacy and their uneasiness with the traditional structure of office visits. Culturally sensitive counselors would go even further toward removing barriers to treatment. Needed services include both general counseling to deal with depression and specific bereavement counseling.

Some projects attempt to help families with AIDS communicate while protecting their privacy. Two readily available and relatively inexpensive ways of connecting people, telephones and computers, can provide youth with an anonymous forum to share information and feelings with peers and counselors and obtain information about educational and vocational opportunities, AIDS prevention, and other salient topics.* Several computer networks for youth are currently operating in New York City, and the National Cancer Institute has been evaluating the effectiveness of nationwide time-limited telephone groups. Computer and telephone networks hold promise for breaking down the barriers that can isolate HIV-infected people and their families.

Support for Grandmothers and New Guardians

Grandmothers and aunts who have become the caregivers of youth affected by AIDS are often isolated by their grief, by the stigma of having AIDS in the family, by their own chronic health problems, and by the effort required to make a home for children, some of whom may be HIV positive. Support networks for these grandmothers and other guardians of these affected youth are urgently needed.

School and Court Advocacy

The youth interviewed in the study need advocates in the school system and the court system. This is particularly true of youth in families with a history of drug abuse, illness, and unstable living situations, who are unlikely to have family members willing or able to advocate for them. Parents and family members may be ambivalent about these teenagers' needs

---

*In part to evaluate the effectiveness of interventions using computer skills, DAS has initiated a four-year study with funds from the National Institute of Mental Health and in collaboration with the HIV Center for Clinical and Behavioral Studies at Columbia University.

and feel at a loss about how to impose discipline at home. Advocates are particularly important for these youth, both to assist in solving the problems at hand and to be available to provide ongoing support.

In many cases, school advocacy is needed to help youths investigate alternative educational settings, such as graduate equivalency programs and magnet schools. Teenagers in families with AIDS require programs that will be sensitive to their specific needs. These can include a flexible school schedule to allow a student to care for a sick parent at home, and a formal recognition that an older teenager who assumes responsibility within the family during a parent's illness may have difficulty accepting some aspects of the traditional student role.

Assistance with Disclosure and Custody Planning

Both of the families profiled in this chapter had great difficulty with disclosure within the immediate family, with relatives, and with friends. Disclosure posed a challenge to each of the 40 families interviewed. Our conclusions and recommendations regarding disclosure are simple: Although professionals and support group members can help the parent explore the consequences related to disclosure and nondisclosure, whether or not to disclose is a highly personal and demanding choice, about which the parent is the ultimate and best judge. The choice should be discussed with every parent, but the right and responsibility of parents to make the best decision for their families should be respected.

Denial of the illness or of its severity played a strong role in the emotional lives of the parents with AIDS who were interviewed. The team grew to understand some of this denial as a constructive coping mechanism in the face of extraordinary pain: it enabled the ill person to function on a day-to-day basis. It also served, however, to delay decisions about disclosure of the illness, particularly to children, and about custody plans that were crucial to the children's security and well-being.

Many social service professionals believe that openness about one's illness is generally healthier than secrecy. Secrets tend to backfire, particularly when applied to children, causing confusion and resentment. Disclosure of HIV status is not an absolute good, however. There can be legitimate reasons for a parent not to reveal the nature of her illness to a child, and a parent's judgment of her child's ability to cope with that knowledge needs to be respected.

When disclosure of HIV or AIDS does take place, it should occur in a supportive atmosphere, in which the parent feels capable of handling the child's reactions herself, or has assistance in doing so. Professionals involved with the family should assess the family members' communication skills carefully before making the disclosure option part of the therapeutic process. Both intensive counseling and a professionally objective stance are essential in any discussion of disclosure.

Disclosure and custody planning can also be dealt with in a group of HIV-infected parents sharing their own experiences. A combination of group work and individual assistance might be the strongest plan. In 1993, DAS will set up groups for 120 parents and adolescents to discuss issues such as health care, death, disclosure, and custody planning.

Additional Resources

As the number of people with AIDS continues to climb, services for families will need to be expanded. At HRA, demonstration project funding provides enhanced services to 600 families with AIDS. These enhancements include caseworkers with reduced caseloads, social worker support, nurse support, and child welfare liaison. This demonstration project can serve only 30 percent of the total families within DAS, however. Although this type of enriched service is vital for family clients, program funding is extraordinarily limited. Demonstration projects can provide important information, but they do not generate the funds necessary to institutionalize services. A steady increase in institutional funds is sorely needed. In the absence of such support, we continue to target services to specific populations instead of looking at the overall needs of all families.

Still Unanswered Questions

Many questions about the impact of AIDS on families with children and adolescents remain unanswered:

What happens to children after their parents die? Because records leave DAS shortly after the parent dies, we have not been able to trace these children. With the collaboration of The Orphan Project, however, DAS is studying at least 200 families to determine who the new guardians are, what kind of financial support they get, and whether or not the arrangement has been legalized.

How does disclosure affect custody planning? We believe that the greatest barrier to custody planning is the unavailability of a new guardian, but other factors—such as denial and disclosure—may be important.

How can we help parents initiate custody planning earlier in the course of their disease? People have to be able to deal with their illness before we can expect them to be ready to plan for their children.

How do guardianship, foster care, and adoption laws and agency practice affect the custody planning of mothers with AIDS? The laws were written with very different family structures and circumstances in mind.

What are the needs of younger children in families with AIDS? Studies of the needs of children aged 8 through 11 are a research priority.

What are the positive coping strategies that empower families to overcome such daunting events as death and stigmatization? Too much time has been spent studying the pathology of families instead of what makes them strong. This is particularly true in the study of minority families. We need to document the spiritual strengths and connections that empower families.

Conclusion

In the second decade of the AIDS epidemic we must broaden our focus to include those left behind. Adolescents in families with AIDS are among our most vulnerable populations, and we must set priorities to address their needs. Individual, group, and family interventions are needed to assist them in confronting their losses and in constructively creating their futures. Mothers and fathers with AIDS need assistance in helping their children cope with their losses, particularly parental losses. Families need timely assistance to create safe, stable homes for adolescents who have lost parents. Communities need assistance in supporting families and reducing stigma.

Either now or later, society will pay for services to the children of families with AIDS. We can either help them deal constructively with loss and trauma when they occur, or we can pay for truancy, unwanted pregnancies, and incarceration as these children grow older. Our study underscores the wisdom of investing in our adolescents' future now.

II

FAMILY MEMBERS SPEAK

3

When the Butterfly Dies:
The Loss of a Parent to AIDS

Ruth Rothbart Mayer

*Ruth Rothbart Mayer, CSW, is the cofounder
of Mayer-Avedon Women's Support Groups,
New York City.*

EARLY ONE MORNING, five days after his fourth birthday, Zachary walked out of his bedroom and shuffled slowly to the living room. My heart lurched. What I was about to tell him would change his life forever.

He snuggled up close to me. "I have bad news, Zach. Daddy died."

"That means I don't have a Daddy anymore."

"You'll always have a Daddy. He'll be in your heart and in your mind."

Secrets

Zachary was two and a half when Michael was diagnosed, in late 1986, with HIV infection. Michael was ill for a year and a half. Throughout the course of his illness, we thought Zach was too young to understand our frequent discussions of treatment, hospitals, doctors. We thought that by talking into the phone, huddled in a corner, we protected him from hearing, much the way we thought he wouldn't notice us spelling words. We often left him to play by himself or watch TV.

One afternoon, after a conversation in which Michael and I talked about his cough getting worse, we noticed that Zach was missing. I finally found him in a corner of his bed, hugging his animals, singing in the darkened room. I suddenly understood that we had been treating him like a shadow in our midst.

The next night he and I sat looking at the flickering flame of the candles we'd lit.

"I'm sad," he said.

"Why are you sad, Zach?"

"Because Mommy's sad."

I drew in my breath. "Yes, sweetie, sometimes I feel sad. You know Daddy doesn't feel very well?" He giggled and squirmed. I told him that even though his Daddy was ill, it was still okay to feel happy. "You've heard him cough. But he can still play with you. And I'm not sick, and neither are you." He jumped off the chair and ran away.

From then on Zachary was heard as well as seen. He got cough drops for Michael, sat in his rocking chair next to the couch while his Daddy napped, and learned to play quiet games. Once, after Michael had an uncontrollable coughing fit, Zachary said, "When I grow up I'm going to have a cough, a big cough. When I grow up and work I'm not going to work, I'm going to play with children."

He became moodier as well. He had a hard time sleeping through the night. He kicked and scratched kids at nursery school, didn't want to be touched, sometimes urinated in his pants because he said other people, not his Mommy, picked him up from school. Some days he said he couldn't walk because his legs hurt and demanded to be carried; other days he refused to leave the house. But around Michael he was compliant and playful, while keeping a watchful distance.

Daddy's Sick

After two or more months in which Michael became increasingly more ill, I told Zach that his Daddy had a bad cough which the doctors were helping him to get over. But by this time Zach had started to act out. I took him to see a therapist, not knowing what else to do as his mood swings and need for attention increased. Correspondingly, my energy and patience were being sapped.

Every night for a year and a half I got up several times: at least once for Michael who was uncomfortable or had to take medicine, and often twice for Zach to assuage his fears.

Children sense things but can't express them. One day Zachary screamed and refused to go into the house because Daddy wasn't working. Zachary's therapist emphasized his need to feel safe. She was able to provide safety for one hour each week: a place to crash toy cars, order me around, have tantrums. But Zachary's life was filled with uncertainty. No sooner had we told him that his Dad was getting better than Michael ended up in the hospital.

Almost a year passed. Michael had read Zachary the book *Lifetimes*, which explains the life and death process to children. One night he demanded that I read it over and over. He got very fussy, asking for dinner, then refusing to eat it, playing with his trains, then asking me to tickle him to death.

Michael came in to kiss him goodnight and Zach said, "I don't like it when you're sick, Daddy."

Michael was uneasy. "Well, I'll get better." Zach averted his eyes, "Well, I don't like it."

"It's like the boo-boo on your knee," Michael said. "It took a while to go away but it did. And I'll get better. The problem is inside so you can't see it but it will heal like your knee did. When you get earaches they go away, too."

Zach seemed more satisfied but then turned to me. "When is your cold going away?"

"It's almost gone," I croaked.

"Use your *loud* voice," he yelled.

I couldn't get sick, couldn't stay in bed, couldn't take naps without him staring at me or insisting that I play with him, feed him, take him out to play.

His teacher said Zach had again been hitting and scratching other children. Up to that point, we hadn't told anyone at school that Michael was ill. Now, because Zachary was having such a hard time, I told the principal and his teacher that his father had been ill and in the hospital. They didn't ask about the illness, for which I was grateful. Instead, they said that it helped explain Zach's recent difficulties.

Zachary became frightened when he got a stuffy nose or an earache. He identified with his father's condition by insisting he take his father's medicine, suck on the same cough drops. As time went on and Michael's illness was more than the obvious cough, I explained that Daddy had a virus in his blood. Our pediatrician, who had been informed of Michael's condition, once scared Zachary when he said Zach "just had a virus." Zach's eyes widened, his mouth went slack. Seeing his frightened face, the doctor realized his error, then explained the difference between a big virus, like his father had, and a little one, the kind kids get all the time.

We learned the hard way how children hear and interpret information. They listen attentively, remembering and understanding by constant repetition. It was hard enough to describe the nature of a virus and avoid Zach's question, "How did it get into my Daddy's body?" (I was not prepared to talk about that), no less to remember to differentiate between a small virus and a big virus. Furthermore, once spoken, it seemed like viruses came up everywhere: on TV, on the street, or among our friends talking casually about a winter flu going around.

Family Changes
From my journal, April 5, 1988:

> My son is confused. Mommy and Daddy don't always talk, the three of us don't have dinner together much anymore.

We weren't a happy family. We each had different concerns and fears. Michael was afraid, his condition was worse, and he was beginning to feel worn down. He was angry that he would die, angry that I would raise our son without him, fearful that I wouldn't keep his memory alive for Zachary. He pulled away, was moodier, clinging to a steely determination to keep going.

Over time, and without realizing it, I became an interpreter between Michael and Zachary. "He wants you to help him with his pj's." "It's all right if he cries, he's crying for you." "He wants *you* to help him." "He misses you, Michael." "Zach, tell Daddy you want him to play with you." "Hug him, Michael, he wants you to hug him."

Zach and I had a future; we could think about next week, next year without wondering if we would be around to see it happen. Once, when I implored Michael to help me look at our finances so I knew what the future held, he refused, saying, "I only wish I had that problem." At Zach's third birthday party, Michael held him up to blow out the candles. There were tears in his eyes. Later he said, "I just hope I can make it to his fourth birthday." He did, barely.

When Death Comes
My brother-in-law, Richard, and I took Michael to the hospital late at night on June 14. My sister, Debra, stayed with Zachary, who was asleep. We spent the night in the emergency room, going home in the morning after Michael had been put in a room and in time for Zach to wake up and get ready for school.

I told him Daddy was very ill. He said the nurses would make him better and then Daddy and Mommy could read him stories. "You know how in the *Lifetimes* book they talk about people getting real sick and sometimes things happen that can't be helped?" I asked him.

"Yeah," he answered, looking me straight in the eye, "like when a butterfly dies, you never see it again."

Michael died on June 15, 1988.

The next day, in his therapist's office, I rocked in a big rocking chair while Zach sat with his back to me, lining up cars and trucks, crashing them, bringing in ambulances and rescue teams, then crashing them again. The room was very quiet, peaceful.

At first, Zachary talked endlessly about his father. He claimed Michael's belongings. "This is ours now because Daddy's dead." He wanted to know where the body goes, what a spirit was, what heaven was. Someone told him that his Daddy was sitting on a cloud looking down on him, which confused and angered Zach. He didn't understand why his father would leave him to watch from a distance. He repeated that the doctors and nurses had tried their best to save Michael and said that *he* wasn't going to die until he was very old.

Zachary didn't really believe Michael was dead. Young children's thinking is very concrete. People leave but they come back. At first, Zach would look up to the sky and call, "Hi, Daddy." Then one day, he asked solemnly if he was going to see his Daddy again. He was enraged when I said no.

Walking to school he told me, "I dreamt about Daddy last night. He wasn't dead, but he's dead again now, right, Mommy?" The dream was in a motel room up North. "We played the tickle game. We were in a motel and we had dinner and we talked and then I woke up and he was dead again, right, Mommy?"

"Yes, some dreams seem very real, don't they? It's nice to have dreams like that. You got to see Daddy again and talk with him. I'm so glad."

Sometimes in order to understand what has happened, children try to visualize the actual death. Zach asked if I had taken pictures the moment Michael died. When I said there were none, he asked if I had one of him dying.

Finally, he refused to do anything unless I brought his Daddy back. He threw tantrums while I watched helplessly, not comprehending the immensity of his upset because I too was distressed, in mourning, and enraged at being left alone to cope with a child and make a new life for us both.

Zachary told his therapist he would never play with me unless his Daddy came back. She asked him if he would like to call Michael to find out if he could return. "Hello, Michael. Yes, hi, this is Mrs. S. and I'm calling because Zachary wants to know why you don't come back. Oh, because you're dead and when you're dead you can't come back. Even if you want to? Yes, I understand. Even if you want to, you can't come back. But Zachary can remember you, can't he? Yes, in his heart and mind and in his dreams, too? Well, I'll ask him. Zachary, do you dream about your Daddy?"

"Yes."

"Do you want to talk to your Daddy?"

"Only on the real phone."

"Well, we can't do that but we can pretend." She held out the play phone to him.

"Hi, Daddy, I miss you. I want you back." He quickly handed it back to her. When we left he was happy, but later he was horrible. The next day he was a beast, but by evening he was happy again. Weeks later he announced loudly on an airplane trip to California, Michael's home, "I'm angry that Daddy had a virus in his body and it gave him a cough and he died. I'm angry."

We moved a year after Michael died. Zachary entered kindergarten in a state of shock. Everything in his life had changed. Although I was still a constant, I was not always a comfort because I was still actively mourning, too. At times I was depressed, angry, feeling isolated and frightened that I would fail in my ability to support us. Luckily, we had family and friends who were able and happy to spend time with Zach, especially his beloved grandmother, my mother, whom he called "Bubbie."

Children reflect their parent's grief. Zach was subjected to my moods, my tears, and sometimes my inability to cope with the simplest tasks. In one of his therapy sessions, he asked why I cried. "Sometimes because I miss Daddy and sometimes because it's now my job to make sure Mommy and Zach are OK, that we have enough money and a good place to live and I don't always know how to make that happen. And it makes me cry." He screwed up his face and gave me a big hug.

In our new home we knew few people. Zach left behind all his friends, his school, his old therapist, and the home which held all the memories of his father. We went through five babysitters in one summer. He plodded through kindergarten with a teacher who lacked the understanding and patience required to help a child in mourning.

He became angry with me because I couldn't provide him with a father so he could be like other kids. Our three-year-old neighbor, Julie, often came to our house to stare at Zach and say, "You don't have a Daddy but I do."

Zach had begun to change in many ways. He'd begun to understand what he didn't want to understand: he would never see Michael again. He worried constantly that I might get sick and die, too.

Some weeks later, Zach came home from school feeling sick. He looked fragile and unhappy. "Come, you'll take a bath and we'll call the doctor. But what's the matter, Zach?"

At first he said it was his ear, then he burst into tears. He wailed from his gut, heaving and crying. "My Daddy's dead, my Daddy's dead. I want my Daddy back. Daddy, Daddy." He cried and wailed. I held him tight, stroking him. "It's okay, let it out. Cry. Cry." Later, after a bath and hot chocolate, he fell into a long, deep sleep on my lap.

Telling

Children who lose a parent to AIDS carry a double burden. They mourn the loss of their parent *and* struggle to understand the illness. Some children may know about AIDS and ask questions about it, but most can't. They either haven't been told or know it's a secret that they too must protect. And while surviving children often feel responsible for the death of a parent, with AIDS the feelings are compounded by silence and shame.

That doesn't stop most children from having a need to understand. When Zach asked how the virus got into Michael's body, my answers were still vague. But AIDS was receiving more and more publicity, especially on National Public Radio, which we listened to every morning. At times I cringed, wanting to turn the radio off or to distract him. It was apparent that Zach had become increasingly aware and in need of clarification, and that led to my decision to explain AIDS after his sixth birthday, in June, when school ended.

We began, on a drive home in the car, what would be a long series of conversations. (I remembered that my father's best lectures were delivered in the car.) There were certain things I wanted to impress on Zach before giving details about AIDS. Most important was for him not to feel isolated by living someone else's secret. He needed to know more about his father in order to remember Michael as a good man who became ill with a virus that anyone could get. Zach needed to know he was a good boy who could feel proud of his father. We talked about how people react to AIDS and how it might make him feel funny to hear their reactions. I emphasized that AIDS was a disease that many people were afraid of, that it was caused by a new virus that the doctors were still trying to understand, and that there was no cure for it.

We talked about the difference between secrecy—concerns that are hidden and reflect shame—and privacy, those matters that many families don't share with others because they are important only to family members. I gave him the names of many people, family and friends, who knew that his Daddy died of AIDS and said they would be happy to talk to him whenever he wanted.

Over time Zach asked many questions: Were fevers airborne? Could kids get AIDS? and, repeatedly, Did I have AIDS?

One day he asked if AIDS could be passed on from scratches and cuts. I repeated that if someone with AIDS got a cut, you wouldn't put your hand on the cut to stop it from bleeding, but you might offer a towel to put on it. "Or a dirty shirt," he offered.

Four Years Later

Children grieve in bits and pieces, not in a continual process like adults do. Now, at eight years old, Zach knows more about AIDS than many kids his age. He's been able to put more faces to the disease—Magic Johnson, Arthur Ashe, as well as people in our own lives. He has told some of his friends about his father, once announcing it to a car full of kids, a couple of times at friends' homes with parents present. Fortunately, in each instance he told kids whose parents I had already entrusted with the information. At first I was startled when the parents called to tell me, but then I realized that Zach was on his own, doing what was important for him—maybe for shock value, to test the waters, or to get reactions.

One fine summer day, coming home from a birthday party, Zach's friend Josh sat in the front seat with me while Zach and another child sat in the back. Josh put on his seat belt and said, "So, how did Zach's Dad get AIDS?"

I was taken aback but pleased as well. As we talked (once again in a car), I was struck by the camaraderie among the kids, their interest in learning, and their support of Zach.

Knowing that the school was going to initiate an AIDS curriculum, Zach brought the teacher a book that explains AIDS to children. He came home that day and said, "Mommy, I know a lot about AIDS."

"How's that, Zach? Have you started to learn about it already?"

"No, Mommy, I learned it from you," he said, smiling broadly.

Zach is not finished mourning; each season, each year brings a new level of awareness of death and loss and a need to know more about AIDS, but having the door open for him to ask and learn has helped him grow. While he will always miss his father and while Zach still talks about him often, he is looking forward to some day having a new Daddy. I would like to take credit for some of this but, truthfully, I credit my son with being persistent and demanding.

When children are heard, they can listen and learn to cope; when they are just seen, they remain silent, and are rendered helpless.

4

The Two Worst Days

Michele Sandra Ramos

Michele Sandra Ramos is a 14-year-old student who lives in New York City.

MY FATHER WASN'T FEELING so well the day I found out. That was the first worst day. I admit that I started trouble, and we got into an argument. All of a sudden he yelled out at me, "Can't you see, I'm dying. I have AIDS." I didn't believe him at first. I begged my mother to tell me that he was lying, but she couldn't.

Until my father died I never realized how important—no, *precious*—his life was to me. He passed away in November of 1992.

My father stayed in a hospice. It was kind of a last stop, and most of the people there were dying. Actually, all of them were. The day my father died—the second worst day—I had decided to sleep late. When the nurse called my home, she asked only for my mother. She wouldn't tell me what was going on. I asked for my dad, but all she said was that my father couldn't come to the phone. She told me to get in touch with my mom as soon as possible.

At that moment I knew something was wrong. I got dressed so fast. In the shower I cried. Not out of sadness, but nervousness—wondering what was going on. Then I realized right then and there he had left me, he had left all of us.

We talked on the phone the night before he died. It wasn't long, but it meant a lot. We apologized to each other, and we told each other that we loved each other. Then he had to hang up.

Sometimes I still don't understand why he had to go. I wish I could hear him, even if he was yelling at me. I just try to remember the good times. Like the time we all watched TV together or the time we watched the fireworks from my parents' bedroom window, just hanging out and talking.

People wonder what it's like to live in this type of situation. Basically, you have your good and bad days. My dad spent most of the day sleeping. I don't know why; probably because of all the medicine he took.

There are no words to describe how a person lives with a person who has AIDS. You do a lot of adjusting. You can plan ahead, but most likely the person gets sick. At least that's what happened to us. You get used to the fact that your parent can't do the things he used to. You can't be loud, or give him really tight hugs. Or sometimes you can't be around him because you're sick.

In the end you feel that it wasn't his time. I wasn't ready to let go. He would always come back. This time he didn't. I planned to visit him on Monday, but he left.

I wonder if we hadn't moved or if we had done certain things whether he might not have gotten sick. It all comes down to the fact that he shouldn't have done drugs. You never think AIDS could affect your life, but it probably will. And you may find you're related to it.

5

Going On

Mariselle

Mariselle is a 16-year-old student living in the Midwest. This essay was developed during a therapeutic session with Lori Wiener, Ph.D., of the National Cancer Institute, who was working primarily with Mariselle's HIV-positive sibling.

MY LIFE IS DIFFERENT from all other kids'. This is because I have two parents and a sister who are HIV positive. So much of my time is spent worrying about what will happen to them. If my sister gets sick I don't know what I will do. I am the closest to her, and she is the world to me. If my father gets sick I will be sad, and I would worry even more for my mother and my sister.

I worry the most about my Mom. She has not been feeling well and can't do many of the things she used to. I can't imagine my life without her. I don't want to imagine my life without her.

But many days I find myself imagining my life without all of them. Some of these days I think about doing something crazy like running away from all of this or taking my own life. When I think about taking my own life it is because I can't handle so many problems at the same time. I am always in the middle of both my parents' fighting and everyone else's problems.

Being left when both my parents and sister are gone is very, very difficult even to consider. Will I be able to go on? Will I still be able to go to college—something I have been dreaming about doing for a long time? Will I be the same person with the same positive attitude? Will I be able to love again like I love my family now?

I don't know the answers to these questions. I just know that my life does not feel fair. I wish it were different. I know I am making the best out of the time I have now with my family because I don't know how much time we all will have as a family. I have another sister who still blames my dad for giving HIV to our mother. I don't want to spend this time blaming anyone because it was not his intention to hurt us. I wish that other people realized how special, short, and meaningful life can be.

6

A Grandmother's View

Ada Setal

Ada Setal is the cofounder and chairperson of AIDS Children Teaching Us About Love (ACTUAL), which provides support and activities for children with HIV/AIDS and their caregivers.

MY SON EDDIE AND I have not always had a close relationship. For many years I didn't know much about his life, but in 1983 I heard he had given me a grandchild. My brother said the baby looked just like me, and I wanted to see her. Eddie was living with a woman named Armida. After Faith was born, I started visiting them more often.

Faith had been premature and she was sick from day one, always in and out of the hospital with pneumonia and different types of infections. I don't know just when Armida learned that Faith was HIV positive, but she didn't tell Eddie or anyone else. Even after she got herself tested and found out she was also infected, she did everything in her power not to let anyone know. I think she had gotten the virus from a previous boyfriend, who had died of AIDS, and she was afraid of what would happen if Eddie found out. Armida lived a lie for a long time. It was a terrible burden for her to carry, but in those days the stigma of HIV was much worse than it is now.

Armida got pregnant again and gave birth to Jesse in 1985. When Jesse was about one month old, I was holding him in my arms and I could tell he wasn't responding very well. He was running a high fever and had diarrhea; he just didn't seem very healthy. Eddie and Armida took him to the emergency room, and he was admitted to the hospital. I asked if I could visit, but Armida refused. I got very angry about being denied the right to visit my own grandchild. After that, I stopped calling and visiting. My feeling was, "Okay, I'll just buzz off." I didn't want to get involved with a woman who wouldn't allow me to see my own grandchild. Only later did I realize Armida didn't want anyone to know about Jesse's HIV status. She knew I would find out if I saw him.

I didn't see Eddie or his family for two years. In 1987, Armida had another baby but this time she abandoned her in the hospital. She gave birth to Angela one night and left the hospital alone the next day. The doctors found cocaine in the baby's urine and called the Child Welfare Administration to report it. People from CWA came to my son's house and snatched away the other two children and placed them in a foster home. When my son came back from work that day, the children were gone. That was when Armida finally talked to him about her HIV infection and tried to explain what had happened.

I didn't know about any of this when I decided to go by their house and say hello. By then the anger was out of me, and I thought I'd drop in after all that time and find out how my grandchildren were faring. I knocked on the door and walked in. Eddie and Armida were sitting on the bed crying; they didn't seem able to stop. Finally, my son said, "Mommy, I have a lot of troubles and I would like you to do something for us." After he told me that the CWA had taken the children, he said, "You know I love my children and I cannot bear to see them in foster care. Would you go to court with Armida and ask the court to allow you to take the children?"

Before I could say anything, Armida said, "There is something else I have to tell you. All three of them are HIV positive."

I screamed, "What!" I could have hit the floor when she said that. My reaction was, "Oh no, oh my God, what are you saying to me?" And then I looked at my son, and said, "Me? You are asking me to take three HIV children? What about my life? I didn't do this to the children. How could you ask me to do this?" I was like another person, literally, when I was hit in the face with the news.

Then I said, "Hold it. This is too heavy. Let me think about this because I don't know what I'm doing now. My life is at stake here." I told them I would get back to them and let them know my decision.

I left with a heavy burden. I knew nothing about AIDS. All I knew was that it was a hideous disease and nobody wanted to get involved with it. I knew that if people found out you had it, they would stay away from you. Your friends would go; it would be like they wouldn't even recognize you. You would be talked about, laughed at. At that time, HIV was like leprosy, like the days when lepers were put in the camps and people ran away from them.

I came home and I thought about how I'd be treated by the church and the community. I thought, "If I take these children, I am going to be isolated, abandoned, left alone. I'm not going to be able to walk out of my house with my head up because there is going to be so much shame around me." I was only 51, but I saw myself as a woman with no future.

I realized that I didn't know what I was getting into. I thought, "Will I become infected? Can I get HIV just by keeping the children in my household? Just by handling them?" I wondered what would happen to me.

I sat in the living room by myself that day, crying and thinking and asking God, "What should I do? Which way should I go?" I thought until I had no more thoughts left and then I heard a voice within saying, "Ada, this is your ministry. These children need you. Are you going to walk away? Turn your back? This is your family. If you don't stand by their side, who else will?"

That's when I said, "God, if you grant me the grace and the strength and the energy, I'll forget about everything else and I'll go to the rescue of this family. Even though my life is going to be on the line, I will do it for my grandchildren and for my son and his lady friend." And that was my decision.

Then I got up and went to the hospital because I wanted to see Angela. I didn't understand how a mother could walk away from the hospital without taking her child with her. In my imagination, I thought this baby must be a horrible sight. When I found a nurse and told him who I was, he said, "You are the first member of the family to come to see the child. Let me introduce you to Angela."

As we walked down the hall, I was holding my breath and wondering what I was going to lay my eyes on. We walked up to the baby and the nurse said, "This is your grandchild." I screamed: "*This* is my grandchild? She's gorgeous. What a beautiful little girl. Can I hold her?" I was laughing with relief and when I picked her up and held her in my arms, I forgot all about the HIV. I forgot everything except that month-old infant who was looking at me, and I said, "Oh, you little baby, you poor baby, you've got a family now. You've got a grandmother."

I was in court three times before the children were actually remanded to me. Armida explained to the judge that she and Eddie were both HIV positive, and told him that they were unable to care for Angela, Jesse, and Faith. Then there was a clearance process in which people from the CWA evaluated me and my home to be sure I was qualified to provide care. Once the paperwork was finished, I brought Angela home from the hospital. Faith and Jesse came about two weeks later.

Faith was four and Jesse was two. They were like strangers to me. Jesse didn't know me at all; he had been only a month old when I had last seen him. Faith remembered seeing me when I came to visit, but she didn't really know who I was. When they arrived at my home with the social worker, they were bewildered and withdrawn. They didn't know what to do or say. I put my arms around them and hugged them and told them they were safe. I said, "You're home with Grandmommy now."

Then I gave them a nice hot bath, a long bath, and got them into the new clothes I had bought. We sat at the dinner table but they were too frightened to eat. I spent that whole evening just talking to them and loving them, trying to make them feel comfortable. When their baby sister woke up, they started playing with her and talking to her. Angela took their minds away from everything else; she really helped to warm them up.

In October of 1987, a few months after I had taken the children in, all three were hospitalized with pneumonia. I was working at the time, and they were spending their days with a babysitter who didn't know anything about HIV or AIDS or how to care for the children. That's when I realized that I was going to have to give up my job in order for them to survive. I went back to court and the judge discovered that I was not being given the kinship money to which I was entitled. He ordered the funds to be released. After that, I didn't have to worry so much about money. I felt a lot more comfortable knowing I could stay on top of things and concentrate on learning how to give the children quality of life. I began finding out everything it was possible to find out about HIV, how it affects the immune system, the pros and cons of the available medicines, the role of nutrition, and everything else that plays a part in the life of a child.

Angela lived to be one year old. She pulled through a crisis in the fall but died the following July, one day after her first birthday. Four days later, I just broke down. I think all the stress, and the love and the energy I had poured into caring for the children caught up with me. I had excruciating pain in my back and ended up in the hospital, but they could never find anything wrong. I was flat on my back for three weeks. In the fourth week I asked my mother to babysit and drove myself to Myrtle Beach, South Carolina, near where I grew up. I thought, "Let me just lose myself in the ocean. When I go back to New York City, I'll go back fresh." I lay in that water for three days and washed away all the burdens. When I got up, I had no more back pain. I drove back to New York City singing and rejoicing; then I was able to deal with Jesse and Faith again.

They needed so much attention. Jesse would jump up screaming and crying in the night. Faith would be breathing as though she were gasping for her last breath. There were fevers and night sweats. I would always pray for day to come because I never knew what would happen at night. Sometimes, I was petrified, thinking, "Is this it? Are they going to die now? Will I be able to get to the hospital in time?" The problems were chronic, and eventually I learned to deal with them, but at first, if you don't understand what is happening, it scares you out of your wits.

I would see Eddie and Armida every now and then, but I was very busy with Jesse and Faith. Armida was getting very sick and she didn't want the children to see her. Her body started to draw on her until she was just skin and bones. She wanted to be remembered as she had been, not as she was beginning to look. I would take pictures of the children to her, and she would hold them close to her heart. She was hospitalized in the early part of 1989 and stayed there until she died. She was just 27 years old.

After his mother died, Jesse didn't cry any more. Until then, he had longed for a relationship with his mother; but when he saw her in the casket, that child changed. He never went through those screaming fits again. No more frustrations. He seemed to realize, "This is my Mommy, my Mommy is dead." When he knew that he could no longer go to her, he began to talk more about her.

Faith started school that year and began to ask, "What's wrong with me?" I knew it was time to explain everything. I told her to sit down and said, "You know that Daddy loves you, but he has asked me to care for you so that you can grow up. Do you understand why he can't care for you himself?"

She said no, and I explained about the virus called HIV and how it shuts down the immune system and makes people weak. I told her that Eddie and Armida had both been infected and said, "Now, when your Mommy and Daddy got together and they made love, the virus that was in them transferred itself to you. So when you were born, you were born with the virus in your system. The same reason why Mommy and Daddy can't care for you is why you go back and forth to the hospital."

Faith said she understood. I told her there was no need to be angry with Mommy and Daddy because they were not responsible for how the virus got into their system. She agreed and then asked, "Can this be my secret? I don't want to tell anybody. Once the other kids hear about it at school, they don't want to be your friend, they don't want to play with you. They just want to run from you." I told her that was fine, it would just be our secret.

I also talked to Faith and Jesse about dying. I would say, "We are all going to die, we don't know who is going to die first. I may die but I don't have to die from AIDS; I could die from something else. We are born into this world and just like we are born, we are going to die. So there is no reason to be afraid."

In February 1992, I adopted both children. Eddie had given up his parental rights after Armida died. I wanted to adopt Faith and Jesse right away so I could make all my own decisions about the children and their medical care, instead of having to go through the foster care agencies, but I was always told, "Wait another year." I even contacted the governor and said, "You have a mother who wants to adopt and care for the children and you are holding it up with red tape. That doesn't make sense." I had to fight to become the adoptive parent.

A few months after the adoptions were completed, Faith died at a family reunion in North Carolina. She had always been medically fragile, but she was a fighter. Every time she went into the hospital, she would say, "I'm not ready to die." Her last six months were miserable. Her kidney and her liver began to fail her. She was in so much pain, she got to the point where she couldn't walk. What she missed most was going to school and being with her peers. She saw that Jesse would be staying behind in this life while she was going to be out of it, and that made her so angry she once said to me, "It's not fair. Jesse's never sick. How come he can go to school and not me? I want him to die first."

When his sister died, Jesse started screaming and crying until he heard a voice speak to him and say, "Jesse, stop crying. Faith is with Jesus; everything is going to be all right." He told me about the voice later and said, "I don't have to cry anymore. One day, I'm going to be with her."

But Faith's death was hard on him. He started acting out and the teacher had problems with him in school. One day he said to me, "I want to die. I want to go where Faith is." I sat him down and said, "Remember when Faith said she wanted you to go first? I think she knew that you wouldn't be able to help me get past her death. She wanted to be here where she could help me."

Jesse looked at me as I was talking. All of a sudden, he was okay again.

Next thing I knew, Jesse was Jesse. He stopped mourning and grieving, and began to help out. He got better at school; his teacher could deal with him again. I think he decided, "I'm going to live my life because that is what Faith would have done if she were alive." He picked up the pieces and said, "Okay, what do you want me to do for you?"

Jesse knows his Dad is very sick; he can see it. Eddie is fighting crypto-coccus meningitis, and he is weak. He has said to me, "I know I'm dying but death is going to have a hard time taking me. I know it is going to win, but I'm going to give a good fight." I tell Jesse, "One day your Dad will not be around. We could go first, but we know he is going to go, too."

Jesse and Eddie are pals now. They talk by phone every day after school, and at night they often have long conversations. Sometimes we will drive over to Eddie's neighborhood in Brooklyn so they can spend a little time together, or we'll drive around the park and they'll talk. I don't interfere, I just let father and son enjoy each other.

When Faith was alive, Jesse understood about HIV and AIDS and he accepted it, but now he doesn't want to talk about the disease. He said to me, "I don't have no HIV. There is nothing wrong with me." Eddie was in denial for a long time, too, and I think that's where Jesse picked it up.

These have been very heavy years for me. It is not easy dealing with pediatric AIDS. It is a mean, hideous disease and a 24-hour situation. You never know when or how a child is going to get sick, or what to expect. You just do not know. You must have patience and love, and you have to give out a whole lot of good energy.

But I have learned how to handle it. Back in 1987, right after Angela had been abandoned in the hospital, a nurse asked me whether I was planning to take her home. I said I was thinking about it and he said, "Do you know what you're getting into? I wouldn't take that child for any amount of money they would give me." I asked why, and he said, "The responsibility of caring for an HIV child is so awesome. You have to have great nerves and strength."

I said, "I think I've got that, thank you very much. I'll be back tomorrow."

7

A Father's Story

Luis Arce

Luis Arce is a real estate management consultant in New York City. Mr. Arce's chapter is adapted from a talk he gave at the meeting "AIDS and Orphans: Unmet Needs in Six U.S. Cities," sponsored by The Orphan Project in June 1993.

MY NAME IS LUIS ARCE, and I have AIDS. Recently I have done away with evasiveness and now I confront the problem head on: I have a terminal disease, and the likelihood of my beating it is as great as that of a snowball's in hell not melting.

This may seem pessimistic, but I am by no means a pessimist. As a matter of fact, I am very optimistic. Every day that I am able to look at the faces of my children is a day of victory against this disease. Every hour that I can spend with my children is an hour of life. Every time I plan for my children is a time of peace.

I was diagnosed HIV positive about four years ago. It didn't come as a surprise to me. As a gay man who had lost most of his best friends to AIDS and was in the process of losing a partner of 16 years, I felt somehow relieved. I felt it was appropriate for me, too, to die of the same plague that was devastating my world—and that will devastate everyone's world, if people don't do something about it.

I am by no means religious. In fact, I went from being an atheist to an agnostic—just in case I was wrong. But I remember the day the doctor told me that I was HIV positive. I remember how relieved I felt because I, too, would be joining my friends and my best friend and lover, if he were to die before me. That feeling of relief did not last long. Just as I was walking out of the doctor's office, panic began to set in. All I thought about was, "What will become of our children?"

Seven years previously John and I had decided to adopt children. We made efforts to adopt children that no one else wanted, and it seemed very appropriate and very natural that we become foster parents to HIV-positive children. We took in as foster children Noel and Joel, two brothers a year apart who were both HIV positive at the time. Their mother had abandoned them in the hospital where they were born. Later, we took in an HIV-positive orphan named Angel. Noel is now HIV negative, but Joel and Angel are both infected. At five years old, Noel has already lost his biological parents and one adoptive father to AIDS. His biological brother, adoptive brother, and adoptive father all live with the disease.

Little did John know at the time that he had the disease, and that he would not live to see his children grow older, or comfort them when they became ill, or caress and hold them when their time came as well. Little did I know that I would face the dreadful task of burying my loved one while at the same time looking for a loving, nurturing home for my little Noel, my brave Joel, and my courageous Angel.

On April 4, 1991, John died of complications from AIDS. He was my life at that point.

Even though I knew about AIDS, and had been to so many funerals, it was not until that day and John's last breath that I realized what AIDS really was.

How would I tell my children about it? What would we talk about? John had been mother and father to the kids. He walked with Noel on his back until Noel was about two years old. In fact, Noel made believe he couldn't walk so that he could be carried by John.

And all I kept thinking was, "I've got to go home and tell the children that John died." They were going to ask me how he died. And I just couldn't think of telling them that John died of AIDS.

Because we were trying to adopt children who were HIV positive, we lived in privacy. We lost most of our friends because we didn't want to implicate them; they all knew that John and I had AIDS. If the child welfare authorities found out, they were not going to let us adopt the children. Caseworkers say, "Don't worry if you have anything wrong, just tell us." But if you tell them, that's when they pull your kids out. That's when they say there's no more support. That's when they bury you. And I refuse to be buried alive.

My family and friends told me "Don't worry, the children are going to be okay." But when you have foster children, they're not going to be okay. The agency asked questions like, "Are you sure you're not sick? Your lover died of AIDS." And I said, "No, I'm not sick." Even if you weigh 90 pounds, you're still going to say no. Then they ask, "When were you last diagnosed?"—they're not supposed to ask this, but they do. And you keep on saying no. I even told my mother not to tell the agency my cause of death if I had not completed the adoption process by then.

In February 1993 I finally adopted Noel and Joel. Angel had been previously adopted by John.

When John was alive, we didn't plan much because John always knew that he was going to go before me. I think John had it the easy way, because he didn't have to worry about who was going to be with the children. I became ill two months after John died. I ended up in the hospital, and, of course, I had to tell the agency all these lies—that I had a job in Puerto Rico, and so on.

I felt, again, "What do I do with my children?" And I think I was probably destined to die that June or July. But the fact that I had not settled where my children were going kept me alive. It kept me going until November, when I again became sick and went into the hospital. Again I thought I was going to die, but still it wasn't so. I didn't have a place for my children.

I am luckier than most because I have started custody and transition planning with my brother and sister-in-law, but I am still not relaxed. Just like mothers, fathers feel that nobody can do their job as well as they're doing it. You feel that nobody knows your children as well as you do, that nobody could give them the love that you give them. This issue has caused problems between me and my family, even though we are very close.

My brother and sister-in-law, whom I love dearly, are the people who will watch my children go to the prom and see them dressed up for graduation. I will never see that. And as much as I try to be un-emotional about this, I just hate it that other people are going to have the opportunity to see the things that I should see.

I will never see my children get jobs. I will never see my children go out there and become something. (I don't worry about Noel because I know he is going to make tons of money.)

While I am sometimes comforted by the fact that I will die before the kids, I also want to help them when they become ill. It's like a Catch-22. I feel like I just can't go through another death—the pain if Joey or Angel dies. But at the same time, I want to be with them when their time comes, because nobody can hold them the way I would. I remember when John died; as comatose and as vegetative as he was, the fact that I was there holding his hand made it a little easier. I know it made it easier for me, and I believe it made it easier for John. And I know my brother and sister-in-law will be great parents, because they have done a good job with their children, but they are never going to do the job that I could do. I've made out my will. I've done everything I have to do, and I'm just waiting. People say, "That poor man, he's dying," and they look at me as if I were dead. But I will not die yet.

I have dedicated most of my life to education, whether it was for myself or for others. I have constantly strived to learn more about the world around me. I think it is important to educate as many people as possible about this dreadful disease because of the many widespread misconceptions about it. We must all learn more about AIDS. All we do is shut the door and make believe that we don't see it—until it slaps us in the face. And, believe me, AIDS is going to slap each and every one of us in the face.

I feel that if I tell enough people about my fight, about the tragedy of AIDS, how it has devastated the closest of families—my family— and how it causes pain not only to the people who have it but also to the people who love them, that maybe even in hard hearts there will be a little more compassion.

AIDS is a tragedy in terms of the number of people that I loved who are gone. It is a tragedy because I see my children going through all this pain that they basically do not understand. It is a tragedy that children should be born into a situation where they're going to die. And it is a tragedy that the forces that be, whether religious or governmental, are completely apathetic about it. I think you can evaluate a society by how much worth it places on its children and on its elderly. In this case, it is very little.

It is a tragedy to feel that you have been robbed of a chance to change something in society. You find out that there is so much you don't know and so much you want to know—and so much you want to do. You just don't have the time.

8

Living with HIV, Living for My Son

Laura Jimenez

Laura Jimenez is a mother who lives in the Bronx, New York.

WHEN I FOUND OUT I was HIV positive, all I could think about was dying. And when I thought about dying, all I could think about was Matt, my nine-year-old son. I worried about what would happen to him when I died. I was so despondent that I even stood one day for hours by a window, thinking about taking my own life.

But I could not do that, not to Matt. I brought him into the world, and I have taken care of him all by myself. I have two older children, a 25-year-old son and 23-year-old daughter from my first marriage, and one granddaughter—my daughter's child.

When I was three months pregnant, Matt's father told me that he was going to marry someone else. She turned out to be a drug dealer. I have made sure that Matt's father can never get custody of him. Matt is very special to me. I have to go on living for him.

When I was diagnosed with HIV in 1990, I had a job I loved. I worked for a greeting card company as a merchandiser. My job was to visit stores and fill in the displays and take orders for more items. I was making good money, and I liked being independent and meeting so many people.

But because of my illness, I had to quit my job. I had lost a lot of weight and had constant diarrhea. My memory was not reliable, and I felt tired all the time. I did not want to go on welfare but there was no other choice. Even so, it took an entire summer to get the benefits to which I was entitled. The whole process was humiliating.

At first I could not handle the diagnosis. I had been going to a gynecological clinic for heavy bleeding. After the regular tests didn't show what was wrong, a counselor suggested an HIV test. When the results came back positive, I was in shock. Why me? I felt violated. The man who I believe gave me the virus never told me that he was infected. I had no reason to believe I was at risk. I'm a good mother, I told myself. It's not fair that this should happen to me.

I practically locked myself away from everyone for the first year. I was afraid I would give the disease to my granddaughter. My second husband, who is HIV negative, rejected me. He would not even touch me without wearing gloves. We separated not long after my diagnosis.

It was very hard to tell people what was wrong with me, why I was losing so much weight, why I quit my job. I told my older son and my daughter; they both have families of their own. But I have not told my younger son Matt or my mother. She lives in Florida and she has a bad heart. I am afraid that the news would kill her. But she suspects something is seriously wrong, and she asks other family members what is going on.

I have made out a will. One of the most important decisions, of course, was who will take care of my son. After talking to several family members, I decided that my eldest sister should get custody. I feel that my sister is the best person to provide a stable environment for my son, and I am secure in my decision. My daughter—Matt's half-sister—will take care of Matt if I ever need to be hospitalized for a short time. My daughter and I have become much closer as a result of my confiding in her, and I was very proud the day she came to hear me at a speak-out on AIDS.

It has been hard to tell people close to me about my HIV diagnosis, but I have gained strength from other people with AIDS. I now participate regularly in speak-outs about AIDS, and I am active in the People with AIDS Coalition. I have a boyfriend, a recovering addict who is also HIV positive. He has helped me without hesitation, and has taught me a lot about healthy living. I have started to go to church again.

Helping women is the best way to help their children. HIV-positive women with children need support groups and psychiatric help. They also need financial and legal assistance. They need love and understanding from their families and communities.

I have taken control of my life. I'm not ashamed anymore. I realize that the stigma was in me, and I am rid of it. I feel good about myself, and I know now that I have a lot to live for.

III

LIVING WITH ILLNESS,
COPING WITH DEATH

9

All Alike but Each One Different: Orphans of the HIV Epidemic

Richard G. Dudley, Jr.

Richard G. Dudley, Jr., M.D., is assistant professor of psychiatry at New York Medical College, Lincoln Hospital Division; and adjunct assistant professor at New York University School of Law.

ALL CHILDREN AND ADOLESCENTS orphaned by the AIDS epidemic share a specific set of concerns related to the death of a parent, but they are by no means a homogeneous group. If we are truly to respond to the difficult issues facing these young people and their caregivers, we need to conduct a full assessment and build an individualized intervention plan around the specific characteristics of the child—particularly age, prior psychological state, cultural background, and HIV status.

Age
Youngsters who have been orphaned by the AIDS epidemic include infants, young children, adolescents, and young adults. They have different, age-related capacities to comprehend the concepts of life-threatening illness and death, as well as different ways of expressing their grief. These children and adolescents also understand the origin and significance of the stigma and secrecy associated with HIV illness differently according to their age.

For example, very young children may not realize that a seriously ill parent who appears withdrawn and distant is unable, rather than unwilling, to care for them. They may then falsely presume that they are somehow to blame for the apparent rejection. It may be years after the loss of their parent before these children fully understand what happened to them.

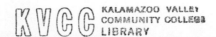

Young children and adolescents have different needs for parental care and supervision, and potential caregivers and child-care systems must respond differently to the challenge of providing supervision and care to youngsters of different ages. Such key issues as bereavement, disclosure, and custody therefore must be addressed in ways that take these age-related differences into account.

Prior Psychological State

A significant percentage of the children and adolescents orphaned by HIV/AIDS come from families that were troubled even before they became affected by HIV disease. They may not have had the nurturing required for healthy development, and some may have experienced neglect, abuse, or multiple out-of-home placements.

Many of the older children and adolescents have been so inadequately supervised that, for all practical purposes, they have been living independently and surviving by whatever means they can find. As might be expected, their lives are often further complicated by other difficult problems such as substance abuse, homelessness, early sexual activity, and even prostitution.

On the other hand, even children and adolescents from "troubled" homes may have had one or more extended family members or other supportive adults who acted as surrogate parents. And some youngsters' lives will have been relatively "normal" prior to the HIV-related illness and death in the family.

Children and adolescents orphaned by HIV/AIDS may also be suffering from any of the numerous other psychological problems, such as depression and anxiety, that can be seen in children and adolescents. These additional problems may make it all the more difficult for them to cope with an HIV-related death in their family. In fact, the need to address these other problems may be even more compelling than the need to address the loss. Any intervention efforts aimed at such children and adolescents must address their multiple needs, or work in close collaboration with other programs that focus on those needs.

Less obvious, and often overlooked, however, are the considerable strengths that many of these children and adolescents possess. Since most crisis intervention models build on existing strengths, it is critical to identify these underlying strengths and help youngsters make the most of their resiliency in their effort to cope with their losses.

Cultural Background

A family's cultural heritage is a major determinant of how the family will make custody and placement decisions, and how its members feel about death and bereavement. Therefore, it is critical that providers learn to help families address these issues in the context of their cultures.

For example, although many African Americans may be reluctant to disclose personal matters outside their families, their definition of "the family" may include an extended group of biologically and nonbiologically related kin. The nonbiologically related kin may have the same rights and responsibilities as biologically related kin, including the right to learn family secrets and the responsibility to protect those secrets from nonfamily. Information about an HIV-related illness or death in the family may therefore seem to be shared with persons outside the family when that is not actually so. If a service provider does not know how his or her client defines "family," he or she may presume a greater willingness to disclose personal matters outside the family than is actually the case.

When helping African-American families with AIDS make decisions about custody and placement, it is important to consider how these families are structured and how they function. The family role flexibility that is often characteristic of such families often means that, in addition to the child's biological parents, there is at least one other adult who already has a parental relationship with the child. A move to this adult's home might be the least traumatic for the child. Even though to an outside observer this adult may not seem to be the most obvious or even the most appropriate guardian, the other family members may favor the choice and provide the extra support required for that adult to assume the parenting responsibility.

There also may be a wide range of cultural variants within any of the broad cultural groups. For example, it would be a mistake to assume that all Asian families or all Asian-American families are rooted in the same belief system or share the same view of the world. Families that are descended from different Asian populations have different views about health, illness, life, death, and many other issues that at least in part determine how a family wishes to manage an HIV-related illness or death. For instance, while some Asian cultures encourage health maintenance and medical care, many Chinese-American families are opposed even to discussing health problems. The Confucian saying "eat [your own] bitterness" instructs a person not to share any personal problems with anyone. This prohibition informs most Chinese attitudes toward illness and death. Therefore, withholding unpleasant information is preferable to sharing embarrassment with anyone, including family members. Since asking for help is viewed as a social failure, many Chinese Americans do so only outside their communities.

To help families manage the issues associated with an HIV-related illness or death in a manner that is consistent with the family's actual cultural values and beliefs, providers must learn to differentiate between *acculturated* family members (those who have taken on the values and belief system of the dominant culture) and those who are *bicultural* (those who have learned to function in the dominant culture while retaining their original cultural identification, values, and belief system). As noted above, how a family manages an HIV-related issue is a highly personal matter that is very much tied to the family's values and belief system. For example, a fully acculturated Latino family might operate out of the same values and belief system held by the dominant culture; therefore a service provider from the dominant culture could base his or her work with such a family on shared values and beliefs. On the other hand, members of a bicultural Latino family, even one with highly developed bicultural skills, will base their behavior on the values and beliefs of their culture of origin. For example, *hijo de crianza* ("reared child") refers to a child who is raised by another family but whose parents have not terminated their rights. While such informal adoptions are common in many Latino communities, they are not legal custody plans. Social workers and other providers must be aware that some bicultural families avoid family court proceedings, which are seen as government interference in what should be a private matter.

HIV Status

Dealing with an HIV-related death of a parent becomes even more difficult when the child is also infected with the virus. We most commonly think of HIV-infected youngsters as infants or young children who were born to HIV-infected mothers; however, the rate of HIV infection through sexual activity, drug use, and sexual abuse continues to rise among adolescents. This population of HIV-infected youths includes some whose parents have died, or are dying, of AIDS.

Of course, these adolescents may not know that they are HIV positive, or they may not even know which behaviors put them at risk for infection. Although many adolescents have reported that an HIV-related death in the family has motivated them to change risky behaviors, some adolescents respond to their parent's death by denying their own risky behaviors. Some may assume that their situation is already hopeless and that it is too late to change their behaviors. Others may act out the pain that they are experiencing.

It is critical that we develop broad-based theories, multiple strategies, and flexible programs to meet the needs of this diverse population of HIV-positive children and adolescents. This is the only way that we can hope to design the specific interventions to fit the specific needs of each affected youth.

Conclusion

There is no question that children and adolescents who have lost a parent to AIDS have shared a similar experience. There is also no question that such children and adolescents have overlapping health, mental health, and human services needs. However, so many other factors describe and define each of these children and adolescents that their differences may be far greater than their similarities. The factors discussed here—age, pre-existing psychological state, cultural background, and HIV status—are but a few of the many factors that differentiate these children and adolescents, and they are but a few of the many factors that must be taken into account when developing a plan to meet the service needs of any individual child or adolescent who is orphaned by the AIDS epidemic. Unless we develop a series of well-conceived, broad-based, and flexible interventions to meet the diverse needs of this population, many children and adolescents who require services will not be able to access and use the services that are supposedly "available" to them.

10

Mourning in Secret: How Youngsters Experience a Family Death from AIDS

Barbara Dane

Barbara Dane, DSW, is associate professor of social work at the New York University School of Social Work.

ALL FAMILIES HAVE SECRETS, some serious, some trivial. Try to recall, if you can, what it was like to be a teenager or child when you knew or suspected some family secret. Perhaps the secret was that you couldn't bring friends home from school because your father or mother was usually drunk. Maybe your sister or brother was "different"—mentally retarded or physically disabled. Maybe you were embarrassed to have anyone know that your mother was pregnant, or that your father had lost his job.

What did you do with your secret? Perhaps you shared the secret with a best friend, and pleaded, "Don't tell anyone." Perhaps you kept the secret to yourself, hoping no one would find out.

What if today you were a teenager with a secret, but now the secret was that your mother died of AIDS? For a few youngsters, it may feel safe to tell; but for the majority, revealing this secret brings rejection, shame, insults, and anger. As a result, sadness and grief are compounded, reinforcing the children's tendency to retreat, deny, and isolate themselves. A "conspiracy of silence" develops around a stigmatized death from AIDS. Such a deception is temporarily effective, but in the long run takes its emotional toll in fear of discovery, anger that a cover-up seems necessary, and possibly guilt.

Although professionals believe that talking about pain and worries is healthy, secrecy also needs to be respected as the way some families cope with AIDS. On the other hand, a death from AIDS can create an opportunity for families to face issues that previously were taboo and to create a buffer against societal stigma.

Because of their vulnerability, children and adolescents who lose a family member to AIDS face unique issues as they grieve. Often they have watched their families disintegrate before their eyes. They struggle to make sense of a senseless situation and to feel in control, even as they confront circumstances over which they ultimately have no control. In addition to parental loss, many experience multiple deaths of a sibling, aunt, uncle, close relative, friend, or significant other. Besides coping with these deaths, these children often must deal with practical concerns such as obtaining food and clothing, and moving to a new residence; legal problems concerning permanence and custody; and other stark realities.

Many orphans of the HIV epidemic have little or no predictability and safety in their lives. Parental death often must be placed within a web of other losses resulting from divorce or separation, drug addiction, imprisonment, or mental illness, as well as a community plagued by poverty, violence, drugs, and unstable housing. Sometimes the result is that mourning has a low priority.

Making Sense Out of Death
Although there is no agreement among studies regarding the ages at which children are most at risk for long-term negative consequences from the death of a parent, early childhood and adolescence appear to be periods of special vulnerability. Whatever the age, however, it is important to determine what the youngster understands about death and to help him or her distinguish reality from fantasy.

Children aged 5 to 8 are particularly vulnerable, since they understand much about death but have little coping capacity. Denial is often a prime defense. Children hide their feelings to avoid appearing babyish. At the same time, they greatly fear loss of control and reversion to an infantile dependence on adults. Often, adults who are unable to express their feelings or grieve openly provide negative models for children's behavior. A child's overt behavior may not reflect his or her true feelings. These children may be perceived as uncaring, unloving, or unaffected, and may not receive the support and comfort they desperately need. Unless children are given permission and support to deal with their grief, they will shut out feelings and engage in magical thinking and fantasy in an attempt to keep the relationship with the dead parent alive.

By the ages of 8 to 12 children have achieved some level of independence. Parental loss can precipitate the reawakening of feelings of childishness and helplessness and, perhaps, a regression to bed-wetting, thumbsucking, and so forth. Efforts to control these feelings result in a facade of total independence and coping. A parent's sudden death will usually elicit much denial and possibly great anxiety and distress in a child of this age. The child's involvement during the parent's illness and dying process will lessen the need for extreme denial, even though some denial will still be likely.

Because anger is a powerful feeling, it may be more easily manifested. Some children may choose to retreat into some symbolic behavior linked with the deceased parent. They may also try to act grown-up in an attempt to master the pain of their loss and deny their helplessness.

Around the age of 13, youngsters may feel helpless and frightened and want to retreat to a younger age when they had a sense of being protected. However, adolescents may be compelled by social expectations to act in a more adult fashion. If the adolescent is expected to comfort family members and care for younger siblings, conflicts may emerge as they struggle to cope with grief and to be mature.

Anger is more easily expressed by adolescents, and it can give them a sense of power to counteract feelings of helplessness. Anger can also fuel depression, however, or be used to punish oneself or, symbolically, the deceased parent. Young men encounter more societal prohibitions against emotional expression than young women. They often behave in a more aggressive manner, testing authority figures and using alcohol and drugs. All these behaviors serve to release tension and gain the attention of others. Young women, in contrast, often long for comfort and reassurance, reflecting a diffuse need to be held and consoled.

At any age, youngsters may not want to talk about their parent's death right away. Children deal with death in a piecemeal fashion, sometimes giving the appearance of disinterest. This is appropriate. We should be prepared to answer their questions about the death of their parent, whenever they ask, even if the questions appear at seemingly inappropriate times.

The case of Lewis (not his real name) is an example of how one child was helped to express his fears.

Lewis

Lewis, a 10-year-old African-American child, had been brought to the Family Service Center by his Aunt Ellen, who complained that Lewis was withdrawn, that he cried when he thought no one was paying attention to him, and that he was clinging to her. She described him as a different person since his mother's death from AIDS two months ago. As Peter, the social worker, accompanied Lewis to the office, he was impressed by how sad Lewis seemed.

Peter encouraged Lewis to tell him how things were going, but the youngster responded with stoic silence. Peter respected this silence, but periodically told Lewis that he seemed very sad. Peter also told Lewis that he knew his teachers were complaining about his behavior, and that his Aunt Ellen was very concerned about him. It was not until Peter commented that he thought these experiences were connected to the death of Lewis's mother that he noticed an overt reaction. Two tears ran down Lewis's cheek as he turned to face Peter for the first time.

Lewis slowly told Peter that he was now living with his Aunt Ellen. In the past, going to his aunt's house had been great fun. Living with his mother in the nearby housing project allowed him to play with his friends, but his Aunt Ellen always made it a special occasion when he went to her house. He talked about his last birthday, when his mother took several of his friends to his Aunt Ellen's and they had a great time playing and eating, and Lewis got a lot of presents.

Based on information that he had received from Lewis's aunt, Peter commented that it was close to Lewis's birthday that his mother became ill. Lewis agreed, saying that his mother had lost a lot of weight, and that immediately after his birthday party she went to the hospital for the first time. He had to live with his Aunt Ellen then. He wasn't very happy because he worried about his mother.

Lewis was in school when his mother went to the hospital the second time. The school's social worker called Lewis out of class and told him that his Aunt Ellen would pick him up after school. When she did, Lewis could tell that something was wrong. He knew that Aunt Ellen had been crying, which was something she never did. She hugged him close and slowly told Lewis that his mother was very sick.

Lewis told Peter that it all started when his mother had a "trans. . . ." Peter asked if he meant "transfusion." Lewis said, "Yes, that's what it was. She got some bad blood then."

Lewis went on to say that his Aunt Ellen had told him that no one could say whether his mother would live. She had assured Lewis, though, that his mother wanted him to live with her, that she loved him dearly, and that she would take care of him.

With help from Peter, Lewis talked about his mother's death. He talked about how cold her body was in the open casket, how lots of people came to the funeral, and how difficult it was for him to move his things to his Aunt Ellen's house shortly after. Empathizing with him, Peter affirmed that it is hard to have a parent whom one loves die. He told Lewis that children who lose a parent always feel sad, and that they frequently have many questions about what will happen to them. He then asked Lewis what worried him the most.

With tears running down his cheeks, Lewis said that he was worried about two things. He regularly woke up frightened at night after seeing his mother, who was very thin, and unable to talk except to whisper "I love you." His second fear was that his Aunt Ellen would die and that he would be left all alone without anyone to care for him. Peter commented that other children have similar worries when a family member dies. Peter offered to talk to Lewis about his worries over the next several months. Lewis agreed, saying that he had not been able to tell Aunt Ellen all the things that troubled him, even though he loved her very much.

"Survivor's Guilt" Syndrome

People generally report feelings of guilt over the death of a loved one, and children and adolescents are no exception. All children and adolescents harbor angry feelings toward their parents, and at times these may be exhibited in the form of wishes that the parent go away and even die. They may view the parent's death from AIDS as the fulfillment of such wishes and may consider the death to be their own fault.

In their attempt to understand the events related to AIDS, children of all ages assign responsibility to themselves for events over which they have no control. For example, a 16-year-old felt guilty because of his mother's death. He told his therapist that he did not treat his mother well, that if he had stayed up with her during the night when she was sick, she would not have died. "I felt I did not keep my promise to her," he said. Another youngster, an 11-year-old girl, reported wanting to change places with her mother: "My mother was in the hospital for a long time. I asked my aunt if I could visit her, but she always said 'Your mother will be home soon.' She never got better, and I sometimes wish it was me who died."

Implied in the notion of "It's my fault" is the concept of control. The youngsters in the above examples harbored the delusion that they caused their parents' death and that they had the ability to bring the parent back to life. Sometimes the surviving parent, grandmother, aunt, or uncle may induce guilt in the child with comments such as, "What would your father think if he were alive to see what you've done?" or "As long as you continue to be bad, your mother will not rest peacefully in heaven." Younger children may fear that their parents' ghosts hover over them, waiting for the moment, usually at night, when the ghosts can harm or kill them in retaliation.

This guilt may not only interfere with the natural mourning process but may also contribute to the development of various symptoms. For example, one teenager whose father died from AIDS reported going on a midtown stealing spree. Unconsciously he was hoping to be caught and punished, using antisocial behavior in an attempt to reduce his guilt and depression. In another case, two adolescents in group therapy reported aggressive acting-out behavior. They described throwing chairs at their teacher and fellow classmates and then running out of school, pushing the guards who tried to restrain them. First, the clinician helped the two youths identify their anger and their behavior in response. Later, they were able to link their anger with the guilt they felt at the deaths of their bisexual fathers, and could then decrease their acting-out at school.

Rituals that Commemorate a Death

Post-death rituals such as viewing the body provide an appropriate setting and occasion for direct expression of strong emotions. Yet children often are not permitted to attend wakes or funerals. Not all emotions can or will be expressed at these occasions, but they can initiate the mourning process. Older children and teenagers, in particular, need help commemorating a parent's death, and adapting to the changed reality. One teenager took special pride in selecting the music to be played at her mother's funeral. Another was uncharacteristically concerned about wearing a good suit and dress shoes, because he wanted to be appropriately dressed for such an auspicious event as a funeral.

Sometimes a surviving parent, or a custodial grandmother or aunt, will maintain the room of a deceased parent as if he or she were alive. Initially this may be a comfort, but prolonging the situation prevents the resolution of the parent's death. In one extreme example, a 17-

year-old girl discussed with her therapist being coaxed by her family to participate in a birthday party for her mother three months after her mother's death. She had joined in, feeling that she would betray her mother—and cause discomfort to her extended family—if she did not attend.

Reunion Fantasies

Many times well-meaning adults avoid communicating to children and adolescents their real views regarding a parent's death. In an effort to offer solace, they may tell them about a blissful afterlife in heaven even if they have no conviction that such a condition exists. This can produce both unnecessary confusion and a wish to rejoin the parent, for, above all else, children need a secure, predictable, and trusting relationship. In some cases, depression, combined with a reunion fantasy, can produce a powerful urge to commit suicide, as the case of Rosa (not her real name) illustrates.

Rosa

Rosa, a 16-year-old whose mother had died of AIDS, was referred to a neighborhood clinic by a social worker. The program offered both individual and family treatment. Rosa's aunt accompanied her for her first visit.

Rosa said, "When my mother became ill two years ago I was not immediately sure what was wrong. As my mother's condition worsened, I learned from an aunt that my mother had developed AIDS. From my health class at school I knew that this was a serious illness and that my mother would probably not survive. I began spending as much time as I could with my mother, caring for some of her physical needs but primarily talking about our lives together and about my mother's childhood on a farm in Puerto Rico. Many of the stories were romanticized, full of freedom, wide open spaces, horseback riding, and a strong sense of community. My mother talked of her disappointment about not being able to realize her long-held dream of taking me to her home, so I could experience the idyllic childhood that she cherished."

Luisa, the social worker, responded that she understood how sad it is when a mother dies and how helpful it can be to share one's feelings of sadness with another person. Rosa expressed her fears of being alone, and recalled the night her mother died: "We both had a good time talking together and reminiscing about funny experiences we shared. I was very sad and cried a great deal at the wake and funeral. There was a good feeling, however, knowing that my mother was in heaven and that ultimately I would join her there. As time passed, I began to miss my mother more and more and began thinking that reuniting with my mother would be the perfect solution for my loneliness."

Rosa was adamant that she wasn't thinking about suicide when she took the pills, but saw death as a way of going to be with her mother. "My aunt discovered my plan and began spending more time with me, shopping and talking with me. I love her very much, but she is not my mother."

Luisa encouraged Rosa to talk about her sadness and loneliness, and to express her fears about changes in her life since her mother died. Themes that reasserted themselves again and again in ongoing weekly sessions were Rosa's feelings of loneliness and her recollection of the happy times she had with her mother.

Within less than a year, Rosa said she was less afraid and that she now found comfort when she was able to talk about her mother. She talks about her mother with her family and friends and feels less alone. When she talks to Luisa she holds on to a locket, which her mother gave her. She now takes pleasure from her school performance and her outside activities.

Rosa's story is a classic example of many adolescents and children who want to rejoin their parent when they feel lonely. For some, the reunion fantasy serves to recapture the deceased parent.

Conclusion

The death of a parent, brother, sister, or extended family member from AIDS is one of the most emotionally stressful events that a youngster can experience. Resolving grief is important to avoiding a number of emotional, behavioral, cognitive, social, and physical problems. Integration and assimilation of a death is a slow process, because it involves making sense of what has happened. For many children and adolescents, loss has become all too common in their lives. The challenges facing families and professionals working with this bereaved population are enormous. Immediate and timely interventions can mitigate some of the negative, lifelong responses to this overwhelming trauma.

Families dealing with HIV and death are often reluctant to turn to traditional community mental health sources for counseling. Secrecy, shame, and stigma are powerful in themselves, let alone coupled with financial troubles, housing difficulties, and institutionalized racism.

To engage adolescents and children in treatment after the death of a parent, we must reach out during the parent's illness and work with the entire family, including extended family members. This type of intervention alone can help families feel safe to say the word "AIDS" without looking over their shoulders to see who is listening.

11

Family Concerns about Confidentiality and Disclosure

Sallie Perryman

Sallie Perryman is a special assistant to the director of policy at the New York State AIDS Institute, New York City.

A NURSE LEARNS at the clinic where she works that a man who belongs to her church is infected with HIV. In her efforts to encourage support, she tells their pastor about the diagnosis. The pastor tells the congregation that one of their members has AIDS. Before long, the whole congregation and the members of their families know the man's name. The man, a father, has not yet told his children about his diagnosis.

The mother of an HIV-infected child is afraid to disclose her own diagnosis and that of her child to teachers and school administrators. Her husband died of AIDS, and he lost his job when his employer found out that he was HIV positive. She gets up in the middle of the night to give her child medication to avoid having to administer it during school hours.

Information has power. Personal medical information developed to benefit an individual also has the power to harm if it falls into the hands of unauthorized people. Although this is true of information about many medical conditions, the dangers are seen most clearly in the case of AIDS.

Families in the HIV Epidemic

Families are often ill equipped to deal with the traumas of death and disease that assault them in the HIV epidemic. The public health system was not designed as a family-centered institution, nor are care systems that focus on an individual patient comprehensive or fluid enough to meet the myriad needs of families undergoing multiple traumas. The specific needs of individual family members do not always mesh easily with those of others in the family. Therefore, individuals making provisions for their families need to establish relationships with service providers that are built on trust and a mutual concern for the entire family's welfare. In reality, however, families in AIDS-affected communities are wary about accessing care, because for them, any provider-patient relationship is likely to be burdened with apprehension, suspicion, and mistrust.

The need for legal protection for those seeking HIV-related health care stems from discrimination that existed prior to this epidemic. The history of biased relationships between people of color and the health care system has been documented extensively,[1] and HIV infection occurs at disproportionate rates in communities of color. Moreover, current studies of attitudes of health care providers toward people with HIV/AIDS do little to assure patients that their provider has their best interests in mind. These studies indicate that many physicians, regardless of race, prefer not to treat HIV-infected substance abusers,[2] and that many medical students are unwilling to treat HIV-positive patients.[3] Yet another study has indicated that evidence of HIV seropositivity or the perception of HIV infection may influence clinical decision making.[4]

The perception that existing health systems have little or no interest in providing adequate health care to persons of low socioeconomic status, to those who are politically disenfranchised, and to people of color creates a barrier to health care for many people with HIV infection. For this reason, among others, New York State enacted its HIV testing and confidentiality law in 1989. The law was passed to ensure that, in the absence of a cure, persons who come forth to be tested for HIV will be legally protected against breaches of confidentiality that may result in discrimination and devastating repercussions for people with HIV and their families. In my experience, persons in the middle and upper socioeconomic classes tend to be more concerned about the material benefits they risk losing, while those at the lower socioeconomic spectrums tend to fear the loss of social interaction and acceptance.

Although law alone cannot overcome all the obstacles to care and acceptance that have built up over generations of neglect, without the law's protection of confidentiality the success of any voluntary testing program would be in jeopardy and the effectiveness of any system of health and social services would be compromised.

New York State's HIV Testing and Confidentiality Law

Article 27F of the New York State Public Health Law specifically prohibits health care and social service providers in New York State from disclosing HIV-related information without specific written authorization.

Informed Consent and Counseling

In addition to prohibiting disclosure, the law requires written informed consent prior to testing, and mandates pretest and posttest counseling. Informed consent to HIV testing requires that an individual understand the value, purpose, and limitations of the test; the test procedure; and the benefits of early diagnosis. The person must also be informed of the availability of anonymous testing, and of the difference between anonymous and confidential testing.* The names of people who will have legal access to the HIV-related information once the test is completed must also be provided.

Other elements of pretest counseling include:

- an explanation of the nature of HIV and AIDS

- a discussion of the modes of HIV transmission, and of risk-reduction practices

- an assessment of behaviors that may put the patient at risk

- an assessment of obstacles that may hinder the patient's ability to practice risk reduction

- an assessment of the patient's coping ability

In addition, the law requires that every person who is tested receive posttest counseling, regardless of the test results. At this session, the counselor clarifies the meaning of the information on modes of HIV transmission and on risk-reduction methods to prevent transmission. In the case of a positive test result, the counselor emphasizes medical treatment and stresses the need to notify sexual or drug-using contacts who may have been put at risk. In the case of a negative test result, the counselor stresses risk reduction and the importance of avoiding infection.

Anonymous testing is conducted at several New York State and New York City sites; individuals are given number codes to receive the test results without revealing their names. *Confidential testing* is conducted in medical settings where names are recorded and test results are protected under the confidentiality law.

Disclosure

The law sets strict limits on every health care or social service provider who obtains HIV-related information. Disclosure is permitted to the *protected individual* (the person to whom the information pertains) and to *people who have been specifically authorized, in writing, by the protected individual.* This authorization must include the date, the person to whom the information may be disclosed, the specific purpose for which this information is being disclosed, and the time period during which this information can be released. Whenever HIV-related information is released to anyone other than the protected individual, such disclosure must be followed by a written statement that the information is confidential and protected by law. A general release of medical information is *not* acceptable for the release of HIV-related information.

A physician can disclose HIV-related information to a *parent* when disclosure is medically necessary to provide timely care and treatment to a protected child, unless such disclosure is not in the best interest of the child or unless the child has legal authority to consent to health care (such as in the cases of abused children and emancipated youth). A physician can also notify a *needle-sharing or a sexual contact* of an HIV-infected patient if that physician believes the notification is medically appropriate and that there is significant risk of infection to the partner. Prior to notification of a contact, however, the law requires that the protected individual be counseled about the need for notification, and the physician must have reason to believe that the person will not notify his or her contacts independently. Moreover, before notifying the contacts, a physician must notify the protected individual and let him or her choose whether the physician or a public health official should make the notification. In either case, the law specifically prohibits disclosure of the protected individual's identity.

Article 27F of the Public Health Law specifies the other people to whom HIV-related information may be released without the protected individual's written authorization:

- employees of health care facilities, when information is necessary for billing or third-party reimbursement

- officials who audit or inspect medical records or to whom disclosure is mandated by federal, state, county, or local laws

- recipients of court-ordered disclosures (these disclosures include a requirement that the protected individual be afforded an opportunity to present written or oral evidence)

- adoption or foster care agencies

- employees of parole and probation agencies (under limited circumstances)

- medical directors of local correctional facilities, and employees of the Commission on Correction

- health care providers who use human tissue in medical education, research, therapy, or transplantation

Beyond the Law

New York State's confidentiality law, although strong, does not resolve all the issues of confidentiality that affect people with HIV infection. Conflicts still exist between the benefits of disclosure and the potential for stigma and discrimination. For example, how might a mother's HIV status on the chart of her newborn affect the care rendered to that infant? Will he or she receive optimal care or will the care be influenced by the possibility of HIV transmission from the mother? One study has suggested that physicians might treat such infants less aggressively.[4] Even if there are benefits to the infant from early intervention for HIV infection, how does one weigh these benefits against the possible stigma to both the child and mother? And how does a mother of an HIV-infected school child ensure her child's access to care, without risking disclosure or inappropriate placement in a special education program? Or conversely, how does a mother move her child from the mainstream curriculum into programs that are specially tailored for students with developmental disabilities, regardless of diagnosis?

To serve clients facing conflicts like these, providers must work toward sensitive, realistic policies that acknowledge the complex individual, familial, and social issues that accompany a diagnosis of HIV infection. An institution's dynamics, like a family's, have a bearing on the handling of HIV-related information, and on the treatment of people who are infected with the virus. These institutional dynamics stem from political and financial responses to the HIV epidemic. Within this climate, a hospital administration that is sensitive to issues of stigmatization may seek creative ways to protect HIV-positive patients from discrimination by staff or even other patients. Financial incentives, such as enhanced rates for HIV-related services, may encourage the provision of services. At the same time, however, these incentives, which require identification of the patient's HIV status, may counter the innovation being fostered to protect the patient's confidentiality.

The social and economic status of people within the institution also has a bearing on the confidential handling of HIV-related information, and must be taken into account. An HIV-positive physician's concerns about discrimination may differ from those of an uninfected lab technician. A hospital cleaning attendant who wants to know the HIV status of every patient on the ward he cleans has a different perspective from the HIV-positive patient who fears that disclosure could jeopardize her living arrangements when she leaves the hospital.

The issues of confidentiality that surround HIV/AIDS are more complex than any law can ever address. Among people with a longstanding distrust of the health care system, the law alone may not overcome a reluctance to be tested, to seek care, and to make provisions for their dependent children. In the economic, social, and political atmosphere surrounding the HIV epidemic, only humane, just, and meaningful interventions will make a difference.

Notes

1. See, for example, Jones, S. *Race Prejudice and Health Care: The Lessons of the Tuskegee Syphilis Experiment and Critical Condition: African Americans in the Health Care System (A Dual Conference Report)* (Minneapolis: Illusion Theater, Urban Coalition, and the Center for Biomedical Ethics at the University of Minnesota, June 1991 and March 1992). See also Council on Ethical and Judicial Affairs. "Black-White Disparities in Health Care," *Journal of the American Medical Association* 263 (1990):2344-2346; and Nsiah-Jefferson, L. "Reproductive Laws, Women of Color, and Low-Income Women," in *Reproductive Laws for the 1990's, A Briefing Handbook,* S. Cohen and N. Taub, eds. (Clifton, NJ: Humana Press, 1989).

2. Gerbert, B; Maguire, B.T.; Bleecker, T.; et al. "Primary Care Physicians and AIDS: Attitudinal and Structural Barriers to Care," *Journal of the American Medical Association* 266 (1991):2837-2842.

3. Ness, R.B.; Kelly, J.V.; Killian, C.D. "House Staff Recruitment to Municipal and Voluntary New York City Residency Programs During the AIDS Epidemic," *Journal of the American Medical Association* 266 (1991):2843-2846.

4. Levin, B.W.; Driscoll, J.M.; Fleischman, A.R. "Treatment Choice for Infants in the Neonatal Intensive Care Unit at Risk for AIDS," *Journal of the American Medical Association* 265 (1991):2976-2981.

12

Custody and Placement: The Legal Issues

Mildred Pinott

Mildred Pinott, Esq., is a staff attorney at the Community Law Offices of the Legal Aid Society. She works primarily in the Legal Aid/ Montefiore Medical Center HIV/AIDS Representation Project,* which provides hospital-based legal services to people infected with HIV and people with AIDS.

ONE OF THE MOST difficult and painful realizations for a mother to face is the possibility that she will not have the opportunity to care for her children and help them grow to maturity. Most of the people I see in my work are HIV-infected women of color aged 18 to 60, although I see many men in the same situation. The parents among my clients typically report that the worst consequence of their illness is that they may not survive to see their children grow up, and therefore must decide who will parent their children in the event of serious illness or death.

Encouraging Planning

Parents often resist discussions about future planning. To them, even thinking about such decisions translates into "I am going to die," or "I am giving up," or "I am giving in to this illness." As a result, despite a parent's understanding of the wisdom of this kind of planning, she or he will put it off.

---

*The Legal Aid/Montefiore Medical Center HIV/AIDS Representation Project is funded by the New York State AIDS Institute.

Sometimes parents rationalize the delay by telling themselves that they feel well and cannot imagine the need for such planning. Many are asymptomatic, and some have never been hospitalized or had an opportunistic infection. Sometimes they don't want to deal with their illness; they are frightened, and confronting these decisions simply scares them more. Sometimes parents think that because they have supportive family and friends, they do not need to document their wishes or take any legal action. Sometimes they want to shield their children from their illness; they shy away from making decisions to avoid having to tell their teenager or 10-year-old that maybe someone else will have to take care of him or her. Nevertheless, if one is straightforward and sensitive to the parent's fears and concerns, one can bring up the subject.

Future planning for children is not only a concern for parents who are HIV positive. All parents should have a legally executed plan of action to empower someone to take care of their children if something happens to them. What if the parent were in a car accident, or were injured on the job? What if a physically healthy parent suffered a mental breakdown? All parents should think about this issue and, at the very least, document their wishes in writing.

Knowing when and how to initiate the discussion is often hard to gauge. Parents should not be frightened into future planning. They should not be threatened with the possibility, for example, that the Child Welfare Administration (CWA) will remove their children if they do not make future planning decisions. They should not be frightened into believing that their children will become wards of the state if no finalized legal arrangements have been made for them.

Most parents need to be guided, as gently and persuasively as possible, to decide realistically who would be the most appropriate guardian for their children. They should be presented with all the relevant legal options and allowed time to think things over. Sometimes weeks, months, or years pass before I hear from a client after an initial meeting. But I respect that parent's period of reflection and analysis. The length of time involved in this decision-making process is related to its difficult, sensitive, and personal nature.

If the parent is not in a crisis, there is time for reflection and careful consideration. However, even if a crisis develops and the parent's health is deteriorating, the decision is still the parent's to make, and should not be forced—although some prodding may be helpful and necessary. Even then, service providers should not make the provision of services contingent on the parent making a decision. Well-meaning service providers can alienate parents by rushing them, or even by appearing to rush them, into making such decisions. Moreover, these hasty decisions can backfire; the parents may later regret them and desire changes.

It is critical that parents include their children in planning for their care. Nothing is more alienating to children than realizing that adults are making decisions about them and around them, but without them. Children have essential input to provide. Sometimes they can signal parents about potential problems with a prospective guardian; sometimes they have preferences about who they would like to live with if their parents are not available.

Parents should do their best to engage in honest, open discussions with their children about their future care as often as possible. Children, adolescents, and young adults have opinions and they want to be heard. Parents and service providers should listen to them, share concerns with them, and allow for their concerns. Children feel less helpless when they are involved in planning for their future care. This empowerment is especially valuable for children who are dealing with the difficult prospect of losing one or both of their parents.

Parents should also remember that children have a voice in the judicial process, and can affect the outcome of a legal proceeding. For example, a child 14 years old or older has the right to oppose or consent to the choice of a guardian, and generally children are entitled to a court-appointed law guardian to represent their interests in court.

Sometimes parents are reluctant to initiate a legal proceeding for the future care of their children because they fear the possibility and ramifications of being compelled to disclose the nature of their illness. They may not have informed their children, other relatives, or the prospective guardians, whether relatives or nonrelatives, about their diagnosis. Many parents fear that a judge or court personnel will treat them differently if their illness is disclosed. They fear that there may be further disclosure, which may subject their children to stigma or discrimination. These are all valid concerns and should be addressed to the satisfaction of the parent before a proceeding is commenced.

The decision about when and to whom to disclose is the parents' to make. At a minimum, parents should be encouraged to alert the prospective guardian, and the children, that the legal steps being taken to safeguard the children's future care are necessary because the parent has a medical condition that may make him or her unavailable. The exact nature of the illness need not be mentioned. The parent should be aware, however, that his or her medical condition is likely to become an issue; in most cases it is the basis for bringing the proceeding in the first place. It is only fair that a prospective guardian be told that it is a real possibility that he or she may be assuming a child's care sometime in the near future.

Typically, it is unnecessary to state the exact nature of a parent's illness in the documents initially filed with a court. Parents must specifically authorize disclosure in writing. In most instances, the language used in court documents simply states that a parent is suffering from a terminal illness from which she or he is not expected to recover. Although that language does not preclude a judge from inquiring further about the nature of the parent's illness, most judges do not. To the judiciary's credit, over the past few years judges and court personnel have become more sensitive to the issues that these cases present.

Family Law: General Points

Parents are the natural guardians of their children by virtue of common law; that is, a parent's guardianship rights are not conferred by statute but exist as a result of long legal experience. Barring extraordinary circumstances such as persistent neglect, abuse, abandonment, or unfitness, both parents have an equal right to the custody and care of their children. Even a noncustodial or absent parent is legally entitled to notice of any judicial proceeding that may compromise his or her parental rights. That parent may also be entitled to visitation with the child. Before a biological father can assert his rights as a parent to a child born out of wedlock, however, he must first establish paternity and be adjudicated the father of the child by a court of competent jurisdiction, such as the Family Court or the Supreme Court.

Legal Options

A legal guardian is someone legally responsible and legally empowered to make day-to-day decisions concerning a child (Exhibit 12-1). A parent can designate a guardian for his or her child or children by any of the following mechanisms:

Wills

A last will and testament is useful when the parent does not want to transfer guardianship rights to another individual until death. The will must be probated in Surrogate's Court by the executor—who may or may not be

Exhibit 12-1
Defining Custody and Guardianship

"Custody" and "guardianship" are extremely elastic terms. Both imply generally that someone has day-to-day decision-making authority concerning a child. Custody connotes the physical care and control of a child. Guardianship does not necessarily require the physical care and control of a child.

A legal guardian of the *person* of a minor is legally vested with the power and charged with the responsibility of taking care of a minor until the minor reaches the age of 18. A legal guardian of the *property* of a minor is legally empowered to manage the property of the minor until she or he reaches the age of 18. Someone can, but need not, be the legal guardian of both the person and the property of a minor. Therefore, a child could technically have one person as his legal guardian and be in that person's physical custody and have another guardian responsible for managing his property.

Parents, typically, are the only individuals who have legal standing to maintain or transfer physical custody of their child, unless the child is in the custody of the Commissioner of Social Services. If both parents are deceased, no one has standing to initiate a custody proceeding. A guardianship proceeding is the only available legal proceeding to assume responsibility for a child.

The Surrogate's Courts of the State of New York have jurisdiction, or the power to entertain, guardianship proceedings for both the person and the property of a minor. The Family Courts of the State of New York have limited jurisdiction; they can only hear guardianship proceedings of the person of a minor and not of the property of a minor.

---

the prospective guardian—after the parent's death. Additionally, the prospective guardian must file a guardianship petition with the Surrogate's Court within three months of the parent's death, or she or he will be deemed to have renounced the request for guardianship. The option of a will provides no guarantee that the parent's wishes will be honored, although the will can serve as documentary evidence of the parent's wishes. The designation of a guardian by one parent in a last will and testament will not affect the legal rights of the remaining parent. That is, without the remaining parent's consent, the testamentary guardian provision essentially has no legal validity other than to document the deceased parent's wishes. The courts will determine whether it is in the best interests of the child to grant guardianship to the person named in the will.

No financial assistance is available to a guardian appointed by will or through a judicial proceeding beyond the regular resources available from public assistance. Children whose parents have worked and contributed to the social security system may be eligible for social security survivor's benefits.

Typically, guardianship proceedings are completed in approximately three to four months because the court requires a report about the proposed guardian from the state central registry on abuse and maltreatment. The court usually requires also an independent investigation of the proposed guardian by court investigative authorities, CWA, or both, as to the individual's adequacy as a caretaker.

Custody Proceedings

In two-parent families in which both parents may be ill, a custody proceeding, instead of a guardianship proceeding, can be initiated in Family Court. The parents can both consent to a transfer of custody from themselves to another individual. By transferring custody to another individual, the parents essentially transfer their rights to make day-to-day decisions concerning their children and relinquish the right to have the children in their physical care. However, the parents' rights are not terminated. Parents technically retain the right to visit with their children and to play a role in their lives. In reality, despite the transfer of custody, parents and the new custodians often agree informally that the parents will continue in their parental roles until they are unable to do so.

A custody proceeding is useful when parents agree on the person to be named. It is also useful for the surviving parent when the other parent has died, and only one parent's consent to the transfer of custody is required. A guardianship procedure still must be filed following the parent's death.

Guardianship Proceedings

Regular guardianship proceedings in Family Court or Surrogate's Court require a transfer of parental rights to another individual. It was the mechanism most often used before the standby guardianship law was enacted in New York State. Usually, the parents and the designated guardian agreed informally in these proceedings that the guardianship would not begin until the parent became unable to care for the children for medical reasons.

Standby Guardianships

Attorneys found that parents were generally very uncomfortable with transferring their parental rights in this way, however. They therefore advocated for a change in the guardianship law to enable a terminally ill parent to designate a standby guardian whose authority would not commence until sometime in the future at the parent's direction.

A standby guardian can now be named to assume guardianship when the parent dies, becomes mentally or physically incapacitated, or chooses to start the guardianship for another reason. (See Chapter 13 for a description of New York's standby guardianship law.)

Choosing a Guardian
Parents should choose a guardian whom they consider to be responsible and who has sufficient emotional and financial resources to care for their children. Service providers should not impose personal value judgments on a parent's choice of guardian. Parents often choose someone outside their family. That is their right, even if there are family members who could assume the children's care. The service provider's obligation is to identify and explain the available legal options, the possible outcomes of a proceeding involving the person selected, and what guardianship will entail for that person.

Questions for the parent to consider include:

How do the children feel about living with the proposed guardian?

If there are several children to be placed, can one person take care of them all? (If not, what arrangements can be made to ensure regular contact between the separated children?)

Does the proposed guardian have room for the children?

How do the other members of the proposed guardian's household feel about this decision?

Can the prospective guardian handle caring for a child who might become very ill?

What if no one is readily available to care for the children? What other options are available? (See Chapter 16 for a description of an alternative planning program, administered by CWA.)

In addition to these personal assessments, there are some legal questions to consider:

If a parent of a 4- or 5-year-old wants to designate a 60-year-old grandparent as guardian, should a younger co-guardian be designated? Can co-

guardians be appointed? If a parent wants the oldest child, who is 17 or 18 years old, to take care of his or her siblings, can she or he legally do this? The courts have been amenable to appointing co-guardians when one of the guardians is either of advanced age or very young in order to facilitate the management of the child's care and respect the wishes of an ailing or deceased parent. A 17-year-old who is not emancipated (married, in military service, or working full time and therefore independent) would not be eligible to become her siblings' guardian until she turned 18. The request for the appointment of a co-guardian is usually framed in terms of judicial efficiency. The existence of a co-guardian removes the need to return to the court for the additional appointment of a guardian if something should happen to the designated person or should he or she be rendered incapable of carrying out the responsibilities.

If the child is HIV positive as well, does the parent have an obligation to tell the prospective guardian about the child's health? If a child is in the foster care system, in the custody of the commissioner of social services, the commissioner has a duty to inform a foster parent about any medical condition that would render the child a "special needs" child. If the child has special needs, it would be in everyone's interest to share this information with the child's prospective guardian or custodian as well. This would enable that individual to care in the most appropriate way for the child.

Does the proposed guardian have a criminal record that involved a felony? The law bars people convicted of a felony from receiving letters of guardianship. There are ways to circumvent this rule, but they are difficult and time-consuming. Sometimes courts require proposed guardians to be fingerprinted; this check will reveal a criminal record.

Is anything going on in the proposed guardian's home that might bar guardianship? Typically, the Family Court and Surrogate's Court will order CWA to investigate a proposed guardian's home. CWA, in turn, will make a recommendation to the court, which the court tends to follow. An attorney or service provider should be aware of any potential problems before a court proceeding. An inquiry is also made to the New York State Registry of Child Abuse and Maltreatment to determine whether the children or the proposed guardian have been named as a subject in a neglect or abuse proceeding.

Finally, since judges have an enormous amount of discretionary power in child custody, visitation, and guardianship proceedings, everyone should be prepared for the unexpected. Three examples follow:

In her last will and testament, one of my clients designated a close family friend and her youngest daughter's godmother as the child's legal guardian. The child's biological father was deceased. When my client died and her friend attempted to implement her documented wishes, the will was challenged in the Family Court by a woman who had been my client's home care worker for two years. This woman had developed very close relationships with all of my client's three children, two of whom shared the same father. The biological father of the two older girls consented to a transfer of custody of his daughters to the home care worker. The court, despite the testamentary guardian provision, refused to award my client's friend letters of guardianship for the child. Instead, the court awarded custody of the child to the home care worker with visitation to my client's friend. The judge ruled that it was in the best interests of the child to remain with her siblings, who were 16 and 17 years old respectively. The younger sibling was about to give birth to a child of her own.

In another case, I advised a 36-year-old mother of two children who was also raising her recently deceased partner's two children. My client wished to legalize her physical custody of her partner's children. She had been caring for the children, 14 and 11 years old, for more than 10 years. Since my client was ill herself, she wanted to ensure that she had the power to designate a guardian not only for her two biological children but for her partner's children as well. My client had little or no contact with the biological mother of her partner's children, although she knew their mother was alive and she had some information about her family. I filed a custody petition in Family Court, conducted a diligent search for the child's biological mother, served her with notice of the proceeding by certified mail at her last known address and was unsuccessful in locating her. I was able to convince the court to waive further attempts to locate the mother, however, in the best interests of the children. My client was granted final custody of her partner's two children.

As a final example, despite a general hesitancy by the courts to appoint young siblings as guardians or standby guardians, a Family Court judge issued final letters of standby guardianship to my client's 18-year-old daughter without ordering an investigation and without waiting for the abuse and maltreatment report from Albany. Instead, the judge inquired extensively of the proposed standby guardian about her relationship with her 6-year-old brother. The judge asked, for instance, whether she had taken care of the child in the past while her mother was ill and whether she was able to manage going to school, working, and taking care of the child. The judge also asked my client whether there were any adult resources available to the child other than her daughter and was satisfied that in fact there were none. Since no father was listed on the child's birth certificate and there was no adjudication of paternity, the fact that the child's father was absent and his whereabouts were unknown did not have any bearing on the case. The case was filed and finalized in one day.

Recommendations

Parents making custody decisions have a range of legal options open to them; however, because of deep-seated prejudices and insensitive practices, they often encounter difficulties in implementing their choices. In order to make the legal and child welfare systems more responsive to the needs of parents with HIV/AIDS, as well as to parents generally, we need several changes.

The creation of transitional, enhanced public assistance benefits would enable families who lose a parent to AIDS to survive the devastating, sudden termination of the enhanced benefits that were available while the parent with AIDS was alive. Programs need to be specifically designed for adolescents who do not have or do not want a guardian; today, these adolescents are lost outside the system.

More generally, judicial education and activism are essential to rid the courts of racism, classism, cultural ignorance, and insensitivity. Furthermore, child welfare workers need training to become more sensitive to their clients' lives and problems. Legal services programs should be expanded to ensure that all who need assistance with custody planning have access to representation or to information that they can use to represent themselves. Broader dissemination of legal information is essential to provide parents with a better understanding of their legal rights and options.

Nothing can take away the pain of planning for another person to raise one's children. But the law, combined with social services and counseling, can help make the process more compassionate, clear, and effective. When custody planning is in place, parents can go forward, leading their lives and loving their children, knowing that their future is assured.

IV

NEW SERVICE MODELS

13

The New York State Standby Guardianship Law: A New Option for Terminally Ill Parents

Alice Herb

Alice Herb, J.D., LL.M., is assistant professor of humanities and medicine at the State University of New York Health Science Center, Brooklyn, New York.

To A PARENT DYING of AIDS, a crucial question is, "What will happen to my children?" Attorneys who began working with such clients in New York City soon found that existing laws failed to meet their needs. Something new was needed, and in an almost textbook example of grass-roots advocacy combined with quick governmental response, something new was enacted.

In June 1992, New York State significantly enhanced the legal options available to seriously ill parents who wish to arrange the future care of their minor children. By amending the Surrogate's Court Procedure Act (SCPA Article 17, Section 1726), the state legislature enabled parents who believe they are at risk of becoming mentally or physically incapacitated, or of dying, within two years either to petition for a court appointment or to execute a designation of a standby guardian to become effective at a future date. In order for the authority of the standby guardian to begin, one of three triggering events must occur: (1) the death of the parent; (2) the mental or physical incapacitation of the parent; or (3) the consent of the parent.

Prior to the passage of the standby guardianship law, two principal legal mechanisms were available to parents who wanted to plan their children's future. (See Chapter 12 for a summary of legal options.) One was the execution of a will in which the parent nominated a guardian and substitute guardian of her choice. The parent retained custody, because the court would not appoint the guardian until after the will was probated; however, there was no assurance that the court would respect the parent's wishes as expressed in the will. Furthermore, the children would be in legal limbo until guardianship was decided, a procedure which could take six months.

The other major mechanism was the guardianship proceeding. The parent could petition the court to appoint a guardian, and then participate in the hearing to convince the court to name the guardian of her choice. If there was no opposition to her chosen guardian, and no evidence of unfitness, the parent could be assured that her children would be cared for by that person. If the guardianship was opposed, the parent, as an active participant in the hearing, could present her strongest testimony to convince the court. The disadvantages of the guardianship proceeding were that the parent had to relinquish legal authority over her children, and could lose custody by means of the proceeding.

Neither mechanism satisfied the needs of young, mostly single, parents whose choice of guardian often was not the other biological parent. Many were unwilling to leave the fate of their children unresolved, or take the chance that a person they considered unsuitable could become guardian after their death. At the same time, most HIV-infected parents, already facing premature death, refused to give up custody of their children. Since standby guardianships were already available to parents of incompetent adults, it seemed reasonable to extend the law to seriously ill parents of minor children.

How Standby Guardianship Works

The new standby guardianship law provides a parent with two options: a court proceeding or a designation (Exhibit 13-1). If a parent chooses a court proceeding, she can file a petition with either the Surrogate's Court or the Family Court.* In either jurisdiction, the parent must state in her petition that she is at risk of becoming mentally incapacitated or physically debilitated, or of dying, within two years and state the basis for this statement. She also names the guardian of her choice. The court determines

---

*Section 661 of the Family Court Act, which grants the Family Court jurisdiction to appoint guardians for the person only, extends the SCPA provisions concerning guardianship of the person to the Family Court.

Exhibit 13-1
Similarities and Differences between Traditional and Standby Guardianships

There are three main differences: (1) who commences the proceeding; (2) when the guardianship takes effect; and (3) the conditions necessary to begin a proceeding.

In a traditional guardianship proceeding, a parent or someone else can petition the court to appoint a guardian for the children. If the judge approves the proposed guardian and signs an order appointing the guardian, the guardian has the authority to act for the child as soon as the order is signed, and the parent usually gives up custody of the child.

In a standby guardianship, only the parent can petition the court to appoint the standby guardian without relinquishing control or custody of her children. The court still has to approve the standby guardian using the same criteria as if the person were appointed as a guardian. The parent decides when the guardianship will go into effect.

A standby guardianship proceeding can only be brought by a parent who believes she is at risk of becoming mentally or physically incapacitated, or of dying, within two years.

When a petition for standby guardianship is brought, as with a petition for a traditional guardianship, the court requests a child abuse clearance from the New York State Register of Child Abuse and Maltreatment and gives notice to the other parent, if his whereabouts are known, and other interested relatives. The court may also require an investigation of the character and home of the guardian by a protective agency.

When a parent executes a written designation of a standby guardian, the parent does not have to go to court. The designated guardian's authority to act begins upon receipt of a determination of incapacity or debilitation and consent.

Once a standby guardianship goes into effect, the standby guardian fulfills the same functions as a traditional guardian.

Source: Adapted from *Standby Guardianship Questions and Answers,* prepared by Brooklyn Legal Services, Community Law Offices of the Legal Aid Society, Gay Men's Health Crisis, Legal Action Center, and Montefiore Medical Center

the fitness of the guardian the same as it does in a traditional guardianship: it orders a check of the New York State Register of Child Abuse and Maltreatment to make certain that the proposed guardian has no known charges against her. The court may also order additional investigations of the proposed guardian's character and home situation. In addition, if any of the children are 14 years or older, they will be asked to consent to the appointment. If a child refuses to consent, the court will take testimony from the child.

The parent must be the petitioner, but she does not have to appear in court if she is too ill. The proposed guardian is required to sign an oath that she will faithfully perform her services as standby guardian. The other biological parent is entitled to be notified of the proceeding; however, within the broad discretion of the court, if the whereabouts of this parent are unknown, it would not be unusual for the court to dispense with this notification. Since guardianship does not terminate parental rights, the other biological parent retains his right to petition the court at any time for custody of his children, whether or not he received notice of the prior proceeding.

If there is no opposition, and the proposed guardian is determined to be suitable, the court will sign an order granting standby guardianship. If there is opposition, the court, as in the traditional guardianship, will make a determination based on the evidence presented.

The conditions upon which the guardianship become effective are death, physical or mental incapacity, or consent of the petitioning parent. The petitioner can indicate which event—death, incapacity, or either— will trigger the guardianship, or decide to start the guardianship by signing a consent. The guardian's authority commences when she receives the evidence of the triggering event—a death certificate, the physician's written determination of incapacity, or the parent's written consent. The guardian's only procedural responsibility is to file the evidence with the court within 90 days.

Incapacity can be either mental or physical. Mental incapacity is defined as an inability to "understand the nature and consequences of the decisions concerning the care of one's dependent infant," and physical incapacity as a "chronic and substantial inability, as a result of physically debilitating illness, disease, or injury, to care for one's dependent infant." A physician must determine a parent's mental or physical incapacity to a reasonable degree of medical certainty.

A parent can forego the court proceeding and execute a designation. In the designation, the parent names a guardian and a substitute guardian. Here, too, she must state the conditions that will make the guardianship effective. The conditions triggering the designation are either mental incapacity or physical debilitation; death is not a triggering event in a designation. The parent must sign the designation in the presence of two independent witnesses, who must be 18 years of age or older. Neither of the witnesses can be a guardian or substitute guardian designee.

The guardian's authority commences when she receives evidence of the triggering event. If the event is mental incapacity, the evidence must be a written statement from the parent's physician stating that the parent is incapacitated, and detailing the nature and duration of the incapacity. If the event is physical debilitation, the guardian must receive a written determination of debilitation from the parent's physician *and* the parent's written consent. If the parent is physically unable to sign, another person may sign for her in the presence of the parent and the two witnesses. The standby guardian must file the original designation, the documents that triggered the standby guardianship, and her own petition for guardianship within 60 days of the triggering event, or the court may rescind her guardianship. If the substitute standby guardian petitions the court, she must state in her petition that the standby guardian is unwilling or unable to act, and give the reasons.

If a parent changes her mind about her choice of guardian, she can revoke her designation. If the standby guardian has been appointed by the court, the parent must sign a written revocation, file it with the court, and notify the standby guardian promptly. If the guardian is appointed by designation, the parent can revoke the designation by oral communication, in writing, or "by any other act evidencing a specific intent to revoke . . .," provided the guardian has not filed her guardianship petition. If she has filed her petition, then the parent must file a written revocation with the court, and the standby guardian must be notified promptly.

A judicially appointed guardian may renounce her appointment at any time before she assumes authority by filing a written renunciation with the court and promptly notifying the parent.

To implement the provisions of the standby guardianship law pertaining to judicially appointed standby guardianships, the Office of Court Administration (OCA) has drafted new forms. These forms, which are available at the Guardianship Clerk's office in any New York Surrogate's Court or in the Clerk's office at any New York Family Court, are relatively easy to complete. OCA did not draft a designation form since the statute itself sets forth a recommended form (Appendix 13-1).

Court Appointment Versus Designation

Because the legislation allowing standby guardianships is so new, it is premature to assess its effectiveness. Based on experience, however, court appointment appears preferable to designation, particularly if the parent is relatively certain that there will be no opposition to her choice of guardian. Judicial appointment provides assurance that the guardian of her choice will care for her children. Even if there is opposition to her nominee, the parent does have the opportunity, as with the traditional guardianship, to advocate actively for her choice. Yet, unlike traditional guardianship proceedings, court appointments allow the parent to retain custody and legal authority.

Designation, however, may serve many clients who are reluctant to become involved in legal proceedings. They may fear opposition from the other biological parent, or feel that they are not emotionally prepared to face such definitive evidence of their impending incapacitation or death. Whatever the reasons, the designation provides for a standby guardian in the event that the parent can no longer care for her children and, in the event of her death before her incapacitation, provides the standby guardian with written evidence of the parent's wishes. A major disadvantage to designation is that the standby guardian must petition the court for judicial appointment at a most difficult and stressful time, when she takes over the care of the children because of the parent's incapacitation or death. Moreover, the parent cannot be certain that her choice will be respected, especially if the other biological parent opposes the appointment.

Conclusion

Now in use, New York's standby guardianship law will be monitored by its creators to determine whether it is meeting the needs of seriously ill parents and their children. It is hoped that the law will make children's futures at least a little more stable, and enable parents to spend their remaining time with their children, secure in the knowledge that they have taken legal steps to protect their future.

Appendix 13-1: Form for Designation of Standby Guardian

DESIGNATION OF STANDBY GUARDIAN

I, _____, hereby designate
     (name of parent)

_____
(name, home address and telephone number of standby guardian)

as standby guardian of (choose one or both) [ ] the person and/or [ ] the property of my child(ren): _____.
     (name(s) of child(ren))

The standby guardian's authority shall take effect if and when either: (1) my doctor concludes I am mentally incapacitated, and thus unable to care for my child(ren); or (2) my doctor concludes that I am physically debilitated, and thus unable to care for my child(ren), and I consent in writing before two witnesses, to the standby guardian's authority taking effect.

In the event the person I designate above is unable or unwilling to act as guardian for my child(ren), I hereby designate

_____
(name, home address and telephone number of alternate standby guardian)

as standby guardian of my child(ren).

I also understand that my standby guardian's authority will cease sixty days after it commences, unless by such date he or she petitions the court for appointment of guardian.

I understand that I retain full parental rights even after the commencement of the standby guardian's authority, and may revoke the standby guardian at any time.

Signature: _____

Address: _____

                 _____

Date: _____

I declare that the person whose name appears above signed this document in my presence, or was physically unable to sign and asked another to sign this document, who did so in my presence. I further declare that I am at least eighteen years old and am not the person designated as standby guardian.

Witness' Signature: _____

Address: _____

                _____

Date: _____

Witness' Signature: _____

Address: _____

                _____

Date: _____

14

The Informed School Project: Disclosure of HIV Status to Public School Systems in New York City

Anne Salerno, Noelle Leonard, Joan Hittelman

Anne Salerno, M.A., and Noelle Leonard, M.S., are former administrators, and Joan Hittelman, Ph.D., is director, of the Informed School Project at the Infant and Child Learning Center, State University of New York Health Science Center at Brooklyn.

EVEN WHILE SOCIETY has moved closer to a more knowledgeable, fact-based awareness about HIV and AIDS, prejudices, fears, and injustices against adults and children with AIDS remain. Some persons with AIDS have been reluctant to disclose information about their health status for fear of ostracism, and families have been forced to fight extended legal battles and confront open hostility while attempting to ensure their child's basic right to an education.

This need for advocacy to protect a child's right to a positive educational experience, as well as the need to increase the knowledge and sensitivity of New York City's educators to the unique educational needs of children with HIV, prompted the emergence of the Informed School Project. The project grew out of the combined efforts of two organizations: AIDS Children Teaching Us About Love (ACTUAL), which is a group of parents, professionals, and other individuals who are dedicated to advocacy and public education concerning the needs of children with HIV and their families;

*The Informed School Project is supported by a grant from the Aaron Diamond Foundation.

and the Infant and Child Learning Center, an early intervention program associated with the SUNY Health Science Center at Brooklyn and Kings County Hospital Center.

Through its association with two large urban medical centers, the Infant and Child Learning Center serves a significant number of medically compromised children and children with HIV, as well as children with developmental delays. The program is unique in that children's HIV status is disclosed by parents, often upon intake, due to the center's work with pediatric AIDS clinics and programs offering research protocols for children with HIV.

To Disclose or Not To Disclose

As the children in the Infant and Child Learning Center approached school age, their parents began to express concern about disclosing their child's HIV status to teachers in the New York City school system. In particular, they wondered whether the schools could preserve confidentiality while meeting the special needs of a child with HIV.

The basic educational requirements of children with HIV are similar to those of all children; however, the compromised health status of these children presents unique concerns for parents, children, and educators alike (Exhibit 14-1). Chronic, prolonged absences; the need for medication during school hours; and the need for teacher sensitivity to changes in the child's health status (as well as to the ramifications of common childhood illnesses) are just a few examples.

Additionally, research has shown that between 75 and 90 percent of all children infected with HIV manifest developmental delays and neurological impairments. The most frequently observed delays noted in school-age children include short-term memory loss, perceptual motor problems, attention deficits and hyperactivity. Because AIDS is a progressive disease, a child may be proficient at tasks in September, but no longer able to recall the information necessary to perform the same tasks in March. Without an understanding of the medical condition that underlies their learning disabilities, teachers may be unable properly to identify and evaluate the educational and emotional needs of these children, and to develop teaching strategies to meet them. This lack of understanding has resulted in numerous children with HIV being inappropriately placed in special education classes.

These issues, along with others, make parents feel that disclosure of their child's HIV status would be advantageous to both the child and the

Exhibit 14-1
Considerations for Disclosure

The following considerations for disclosure have been viewed as important by parents involved in the Informed School Project:

Extended absences
frequent hospitalizations
recuperation periods at home
frequent medical appointments

Educational requirements
neurological problems
attention deficits
short-term memory loss
perceptual motor difficulties
general effects of extended absences
  on educational performance

Health status
sudden fever
frequent need to use the bathroom
listlessness
lack of endurance and energy

Medication schedule
medication needs to be administered
  during school hours

Sources: The Infant and Child Learning Center; ACTUAL

teacher; however, they often fear the social consequences of disclosure. A careless breach of confidentiality can be devastating. Families have been denied housing, been rejected by their neighbors, and lost valuable resources as a result of such breaches. Moreover, school personnel, as well as children and parents, are often ignorant about how HIV is transmitted. Irrational fears about teachers and children becoming infected through casual contact have led to HIV-infected children being banned from school and rejected by classmates.

New York State has a clear confidentiality law that prohibits anyone (with only a few exceptions) from revealing information related to a person's HIV status without the written consent of the infected person or that person's legal guardian (see Chapter 11). The New York City Board of Education has adopted a policy that follows the state law (Exhibit 14-2 and Appendix 14-1), and has developed an AIDS training program to implement the policy among teachers and staff. Because this has been a slow process, however, a large number of teachers and direct service staff have not yet received basic AIDS education nor been made aware of the laws and policies related to confidentiality and disclosure. The Informed School Project works to fill that gap, providing essential support and training for parents, children, teachers, and school service staff.

How the Project Works

The Informed School Project staff consists of a project administrator and child advocates, many of whom are parents of children with HIV, who receive training in issues relevant to disclosure of HIV status. Their initial role is to counsel and support parents as they consider their disclosure options. They discuss the pros and cons of disclosure, as well as the disclosure process and the role of the Informed School Project.

Once a parent makes a preliminary decision to disclose, a child advocate arranges a meeting with the school's principal to ascertain if the school administration and teaching staff have received AIDS training, and to judge whether or not the school would be a safe and supportive environment for disclosure. If necessary, the Informed School Project will offer preliminary training on AIDS-related issues to the principal, and link the school with the Board of Education's AIDS training programs.

The child advocate then meets again with the parent to report the results of this preliminary meeting. If the parent decides to continue with disclosure, another meeting is arranged, between the school's principal (if desired), the child's teacher, the parent, and the child advocate. The child advocate accompanies the parent to the meeting to act as a support, to offer information to the teacher on issues of HIV transmission, and to promote the use of universal infection control precautions in the school setting.

One of the most important roles of the child advocate is to protect the confidentiality of the parent and child. The advocate is responsible for reviewing the New York State confidentiality law and Board of Education

Exhibit 14-2
When Referral for Medical or Social Services May Be Necessary

---

If a staff member believes that a student is in crisis due to his/her HIV-illness or that of a family member, and the student requires intervention such as bereavement counseling or safer sex counseling, the student should be referred for service. The student's difficulty (e.g., change in mood, inability to sustain academic progress, etc.) should be the basis for the referral and not the HIV status of the student or the student's family member. The confidential HIV-related information may not be disclosed when making a referral for services without specific written consent for the release of this information.

Source: New York City Public Schools *Guidelines for Students with HIV-infection, HIV-related Illness and/or AIDS* (Special Circular No. 37)

rules with those present and then completing a special form to record the names of persons to whom disclosure has been made. This form is signed by the parent, witnessed by the advocate, notarized, and then kept in confidential files at the Informed School Project Office.

Once the disclosure has been made, the Informed School Project staff remains available to offer initial training in the use of universal precautions in the classroom (the project provides the school with an initial supply of gloves to be used with all students). The project also offers a teacher support group, run by a social worker, to provide teachers with a forum to discuss concerns and ideas and to share their experiences in working with children with HIV/AIDS.

The Informed School Project is still in its infancy. The first six to eight months were spent in promoting the project among New York City Board of Education personnel and AIDS training groups as well as community and medical organizations. Word of the program has been increasing among parents through the project's work with these organizations.

An initial child advocate training session took place in June 1992. Four child advocates participated in the two-day session, which focused on the New York City Board of Education AIDS training policies, an update on HIV/AIDS research, the latest word on modes of transmission, the use of universal precautions in the classroom, and an introduction to the Informed School Project's policies and procedures. A second training session took place in December, with six advocates attending. Role playing of possible disclosure meeting scenarios was incorporated into both training sessions.

The project has made four successful disclosures so far, two to classroom teachers and two to members of school committees on special education. The response of school personnel has been receptive and positive. Currently, the project is working with a school with no previous AIDS training to increase the staff's awareness of HIV/AIDS-related issues before the actual disclosure takes place. In all cases, the project's child advocates have met with open and honest concern on the part of principals, administrators, teachers, and parents alike. As more parents of children with HIV begin to feel comfortable with their children's teachers, we anticipate more disclosures to be requested.

As more and more children with HIV enter the school system, there will be a greater need for training of school personnel on the issues surrounding the education of these medically fragile, immunocompromised children. The Informed School Project is designed to help meet this growing need within New York City. The project's success to date has given those of us involved strong hope that parents, educators, health care professionals, and citizens are ready to form strong alliances to help provide positive educational experiences for children with HIV.

Appendix 14-1: Commonly Asked Questions and Answers Regarding HIV Confidentiality

Q. *What do I do if a student tells me that he or she is HIV positive? Is there anyone I am required to tell?*

A. No. In accordance with Chancellor's regulations and the New York State public health law, you should maintain the confidentiality of this information and should not disclose such a condition on behalf of any individual. If you have a question concerning a specific individual or situation, refer that question without disclosing identifying information to the Comprehensive Health Coordinator assigned to your superintendency, or call the Office of Legal Services.

Q. *If a colleague discloses that he/she is HIV positive, should I tell someone?*

A. This information is not yours to share and should not be shared or disclosed without the explicit consent of the affected person.

Q. *If a student discloses the HIV status of a family member, what should I do?*

A. You can take no direct action specific to this disclosure to assist the family member, but you can provide assistance, guidance, and referral to the student who may be experiencing difficulty associated with his/her family crisis.

Q. *If I refer a student to an outside health care provider and the student uses the family's Medicaid card in seeking treatment for HIV and the family is later notified of the child's condition, is the school responsible for a breach in confidentiality?*

A. Under New York State law, when a person obtains what is defined as confidential HIV-related information in the course of providing any health or social service, he or she must not disclose this information. There are a number of exceptions to this general rule, including the permitted disclosure to a health care provider or facility when knowledge of the HIV-related information is necessary to provide appropriate care or treatment. Thus a school staff member who acquires knowledge of a student's HIV status through working in this program and who then refers that student for *outside* HIV treatment *would be permitted* to tell the outside health care provider the student's

HIV status. The outside provider, as the recipient of this information, would be bound (if the provider is located in New York State) by the same state rules and limitations. However, the provider's actions in this regard would not be the school staff person's responsibility. If you have any questions about a specific circumstance, please call your Comprehensive Health Coordinator, or the Office of Legal Services.

Q. *If a student announces that he/she is HIV positive and he/she is sexually active, should we suggest condom use?*

A. If the student engages in a discussion, it is important to discuss the benefits of abstinence from sexual activity since he/she is now in a position to infect others. If the student is sexually active, however, and requests a condom, the condom should be made available if the student is in a high school program.

Q. *May staff disclose confidential HIV-related information to their supervisors without the consent of the parent, legal guardian, or the protected individual?*

A. No. Staff may not disclose the confidential information without the consent of the parent, legal guardian, or the protected individual. However, staff may confer and seek advice from their supervisors as long as they do not reveal any identifying information.

Q. *May staff disclose whether a student is receiving HIV-related medication?*

A. No. All information which can identify or reasonably identify an individual's HIV status is confidential.

Q. *May staff disclose information that does not identify or reasonably identify an individual's HIV status?*

A. Yes. As long as the information does not identify or cannot reasonably identify an individual's HIV status.

Q. *May staff encourage that the protected individual share the confidential HIV-related information with others?*

A. Sometimes. Staff members may encourage the protected individual to share the information with appropriate parties when it would assist in ensuring that suitable care and treatment are rendered.

Q. *May confidential HIV-related information which has been disclosed through an authorization for the release of confidential HIV-related information be copied?*

A. No.

Q. *May confidential HIV-related information be disclosed through a request under the Freedom of Information Law?*

A. No.

Q. *Who is to be trained concerning the requirements in maintaining the confidentiality of HIV-related information?*

A. All New York City Public School employees, volunteers who are authorized to provide services, and contract agents should be trained in order to protect the confidentiality of HIV-related information.

Q. *If reports are received by staff members from outside agencies (e.g., preschools, foster care agencies, etc.) which contain confidential HIV-related information but do not contain the authorization for the release of the confidential HIV-related information, what should the staff member do?*

A. The staff member should return the report to the sender instructing them to delete the confidential HIV-related information and that after the information is deleted the report may be resubmitted. Moreover, the staff member must not disclose the confidential HIV-related information which was illegally forwarded to him/her.

Q. *In the classroom, if a student discloses his or her HIV status or that of a family member or friend, what do I do?*

A. First, thank the student for sharing the situation with the class. Recognize that this is a sensitive issue and by disclosing this information, the student has entrusted the class with very private information. Then refocus the classroom discussion to how students can show support for peers who are ill or have significant others who are ill.

   Keep in mind: Don't encourage or discourage the student from sharing. However, be aware that a student may suffer emotionally from overdisclosing. You may want to stop the student from continuing to disclose the information and redirect discussion if the students appear unduly anxious. **You may also want to consider involving a trained counselor in further general discussions on this issue.** In addition, while discussing the subject of people with HIV infection and/or AIDS, *never* ask students *who* they know with the disease.

Source: New York City Public Schools *Guidelines for Students with HIV-Infection, HIV-Related Illness and/or AIDS* (Special Circular No. 37).

For a copy of Special Circular No. 37, contact Administrative Services, New York City Board of Education, 110 Livingston Street, Brooklyn, NY 11201; (718) 935-3225.

15

The Well Children in AIDS Families Project: A Hospital-Based Program

Lockhart McKelvy

Lockhart McKelvy, CSW, is the coordinator of the Well Children in AIDS Families Project at the Beth Israel Medical Center in New York City.

CHILDREN DEPEND ON THEIR parents for the necessities of life: if the parent is threatened, the child is at risk as well. While we know that children whose parents have died of AIDS will live with the handicap of absent parents, we can lessen the consequences of that tragedy. In 1987, the departments of social work and psychiatry at the Beth Israel Medical Center started the Well Children in AIDS Families Project* to address the mental health needs of HIV-negative children living with parents who are infected with HIV or who have AIDS.

Problems Addressed by the Program

One of the most difficult dilemmas confronted by children in AIDS-affected families is the stigma associated with the disease. Almost none of the children I have encountered have risked telling best friends about their parent's diagnosis. Teens report that when they walk down the sidewalk with a parent who looks emaciated and weak, they feel embarrassed and

*The Well Children in AIDS Families Project was funded in its first year by the United Hospital Fund. In addition, the program has been financially sustained by the Spunk Fund, the Mazer Family, United Jewish Appeal, and the Robbins Foundation. The departments of social work and development of Beth Israel Medical Center have undertaken the writing and statistical analysis necessary for this program to receive annual funding.

ashamed. Children experience an intense struggle between loyalty to their parents and the necessity of maintaining, if not status, at least anonymity in their communities (Exhibit 15-1).

Moreover, the atmosphere in many schools is charged with aggression and danger. Fighting is a common expression of self-worth, turf, and importance. Children use the insult of "Your mother has AIDS" as an instant method of starting a fight. Many teenage boys and girls are unable to resist the impulse to fight when they hear this kind of remark.

The roller coaster of illness and relative health that is typical of AIDS as a chronic disease arouses difficult feelings for children and teens. The Well

Exhibit 15-1
How Children React When a Family Member Has AIDS

How Children React to AIDS

When a family member has AIDS, children are faced with many problems:

- understanding what is happening to the person with AIDS (medical problems, hospitalization, home care)

- dealing with their own feelings (worry, fear, anger, sadness, confusion)

- knowing what to tell other people in the family and in the community

- worrying about losing a very important person (parent, brother, sister) and being left alone

How Children Show Their Feelings

Children usually do not talk about how they feel. Instead, they show their feelings through *behavior*. School problems can be one sign that a child is upset. Another sign is fighting. Others are refusing to go outside the home, excessive sadness, or difficulty sleeping. Some children are noisy and aggressive in showing their feelings. Others are quiet and withdrawn.

Children at different ages show their feelings in their own ways. When teenagers are upset, they sometimes show it by using drugs, avoiding school, or getting involved with the wrong friends. All of these behaviors can be signs that something is wrong inside.

Also, children often blame themselves for family problems, even when the problem is not their fault. And when the problem is not talked about, as happens with AIDS, their fear and misunderstanding can grow.

Source: Excerpted from "How Children React When a Family Member Has AIDS," Beth Israel Medical Center.

Children in AIDS Families Project addresses the intense mood swings and the worry that children experience when their parent is diagnosed with a new opportunistic infection. This anxiety affects the child's behavior. Moods and behaviors range from isolation and withdrawal to tantrums and acting out through fighting or other aggressive acts. In this respect the children in this program are not unusual; most children who receive treatment in psychiatric outpatient settings are referred because of behavioral difficulties.

Children who lose a parent to AIDS have a particularly difficult time owing to their feelings of shame and isolation. They do not feel free to discuss their loss in school or with friends. Imagine keeping this kind of catastrophe to yourself as an adult. In addition, some children may be ashamed that their parents were drug addicts. This added shame further complicates the bereavement process. In some cases both parents are infected. This situation is especially difficult to manage in treatment. We are swimming against the intense stream of suicidal thoughts, depression, and hopelessness a child feels when he or she is abandoned by both parents. A therapeutic relationship is slow and difficult in coming.

In addition, some parents are understandably reluctant to make appropriate future plans for their children. In our program, parents are encouraged to make decisions as soon as possible, and, when possible, to reassure their children that they have taken steps on their behalf. This planning is difficult, and frequently slow, but for most children the bottom line is still, "What is going to happen to me?" At a minimum, this process provides some reassurance that the parent has been able to take charge in a time of crisis.

Services Provided by the Program
The Well Children in AIDS Families Project offers a diverse and creative array of free services to address the complex needs of children in families that have been affected by HIV/AIDS. Children come to the program from every borough; their parents do not have to be followed by the Beth Israel Medical Center.

The project was originally intended to develop support groups, treatment models, and intervention strategies for these children; to disseminate results of its work to other agencies; and to educate health care professionals and AIDS-affected families. Fairly quickly, however, it became clear that our original plans needed revising. First, we abandoned the support group model in favor of a family crisis model of treatment. Because of the stigma and shame associated with the disease, AIDS-affected families were not interested in treatment that required disclosure to a group. We focused instead on the issues of disclosure and treatment within the family. On the other hand, we expanded our education and outreach efforts in order to increase our pool of referrals and to promote understanding of the problem among mental health professionals.

To increase further the program's referral base and exposure, and to avoid adding the stigma that can accompany a psychiatric diagnosis to the problems faced by our clients, we moved the program from the department of child psychiatry to a patient care area that served primarily pediatric outpatients. This move also increased our access to the medical units of the hospital, which house adult AIDS patients. Today, I often first make contact with a prospective family in a patient's room.

Parents are offered consultations regarding disclosure. No task is more difficult for any parent than telling children that the parent will become very sick, and most probably will not be able to fulfill what the parent and the family see as parental obligations. In our consultations with adults, we try to help them work through their fantasies and feelings concerning this difficult and important task. A therapeutic relationship can begin with these consultations and can continue throughout the bereavement process.

The program also offers ongoing counseling to children who would benefit from special attention. Services include individual, group, and family therapy; games and art therapy, to facilitate the developing therapeutic relationship and to encourage communication; and bereavement therapy for children who have lost one or both parents to AIDS.

In addition to our therapeutic services to AIDS-affected families, we also provide consultation and information to adult AIDS team members concerning work with the Child Welfare Administration, Family Court, and the school system.

In particular, we are helping families make early and responsible decisions about the long-term welfare of their children. As the AIDS epidemic grows, the need for early planning is increasing. Too often, children become caught in struggles between relatives, almost always at the expense of the child. If I am aware that there is a potential custody dispute between the maternal and paternal sides of a family or between aunts and uncles, I will attempt to set up a family meeting where I can moderate an open discussion. In doing so, I place myself as a step before the difficult Family Court process in hopes of minimizing the negative impact on the child.

Finally, the Well Children in AIDS Families Project is dedicated to increasing public and professional awareness of the catastrophic life experiences of these children. I reach out to schools, speak at community meetings, and distribute our brochure, "How Children React When a Family Member Has AIDS" (now in its third printing), to help professionals and potential clients understand what a child goes through when a family member is diagnosed.

Where We Are Now

The Well Children in AIDS Families Project is providing more services to more children than ever before. While some of the increase can be attributed to the growing numbers of children affected by the epidemic, the effect of our early program changes should not be underestimated. In some areas, however, we have begun to revisit our original model. To enrich the peer experience of the teenagers in the program, and to combat the isolation that can result from the family treatment and individual therapy models, we have started to use group therapy again. This time the co-leader is an experienced social worker with background working with families and children. The group is not an easy one to facilitate, but the results can be gratifying. And we have begun consultations with the program's original home, the department of child psychiatry, for help in addressing the difficult and complex problems presented by these children.

Support of the social work administration has also been important. The resulting freedom of movement has been very helpful in engaging families who may be already overburdened with appointments. By attending rounds with adult AIDS team social workers, meeting parents in outpatient clinics, and being able to move throughout the medical center, I have been able to reach out more effectively to potential clients. And the opportunity to attend special events in the evening, bring art supplies, and give small birthday and holiday gifts has enriched family services.

Where Do We Go from Here?

Looking at the social service system as a whole, two gaps come to mind. The first is the paucity of services that are available to overburdened foster families. Children who have lost parents to AIDS have special needs that foster families can provide, if they have some preparation. In many current placements, however, the foster family has had inadequate support, if any. These foster families are going to require a more comprehensive network of trained workers to provide ongoing counseling, crisis intervention, and advocacy within the school and probate systems.

Finally, the children who are suffering through the AIDS epidemic must be followed and studied. We have an opportunity to use funding allocated to the AIDS epidemic for long-term evaluation of these children. Such long-term study could indicate an optimal model for treatment and point out these children's developmental pitfalls. The increased understanding that we gain through such research will better prepare us as clinicians to meet the complex challenges presented by these young survivors.

16

The Child Welfare Administration's Early Permanency Planning Project

Regina J. Prince is the director of the New York City Child Welfare Administration's Special Projects Unit.

AIDS CASTS A DARK and frightening cloud over a family's future. The surviving children must be placed in someone's care, and parents who have no family or friends to assume guardianship of their children worry about the children they will leave behind. The knowledge that they might not be able to provide their children with care, comfort, and love can be too painful for parents to bear, leaving them feeling helpless and angry. Their children fear abandonment, and worry about who will care for them if their parent dies.

Over the past few years, parents with HIV have started to ask the New York City Child Welfare Administration (CWA) about preparing a foster home for their children before placement actually becomes necessary. These parents want to care for their children for as long as they are able, and at the same time know exactly where their children will go when they enter foster care.

In response to these requests, CWA developed a pilot program, the Early Permanency Planning Project, to identify foster homes for children of parents with HIV illness while the children are still living at home. The Early Permanency Planning Project represents an initial step toward empowering parents with HIV to play an instrumental role in developing permanent plans for their children. By encouraging the parent to participate in recreational activities with his or her children and the targeted foster parents, and by allowing the children to be placed with the foster parents during periods of crisis and then returned home, the program promotes a supportive, gradual transition based on a trusting relationship between the biological and foster families.

By April 1993, the Early Permanency Planning Project was serving 80 families with 209 children. While the full size of the target population has not been established, the current caseload is only a small fraction of the total population in need. The Early Permanency Planning Project is operated entirely through established city and voluntary child care agency program budgets adopted for other purposes.

Eligibility

The Early Permanency Planning Project is designed for families in which the parent or parents are HIV positive and symptomatic, and in which there are no ex-spouses, relatives, friends, or others able to assume legal guardianship of the children. The project is limited to families who will likely need foster care services within six months. Eligible parents fall into two distinct groups:

- parents with a relative or friend willing to care for the child by becoming a foster parent, but unable to become the legal guardian because of the service needs of the family or for other reasons (not to be confused with kinship foster care, which is available only in cases of abuse or neglect)

- parents without a relative or friend to care for their children, and who want CWA to recruit a foster home

The majority of the parents participating in the project are already receiving services from a service provider—the New York City Human Resources Administration's Division of AIDS Services, a purchased preventive service program, a hospital-based program, or some other agency or program. In most cases, this provider makes the initial contact with CWA. Since only those families who are willing to place their children with CWA are eligible for the Early Permanency Planning Project, providers should determine whether parents are truly likely to place their children in foster care before referring them. In particular, providers should thoroughly explore the family's resources to determine that there are no relatives able to assume custody of the children.

How the Process Works

The parent or service provider first contacts the director of the CWA Special Projects Unit or the Early Permanency Planning Project Manager. Typical information that is required to enter the project is listed in Exhibit 16-1. If the initial contact is by phone, a follow-up letter is recommended. The parent or service provider must indicate whether the parent intends to have CWA place his or her children with a friend or relative willing to act as a foster parent. Service providers should contact any potential foster parent proposed by the parent and confirm that he or she has agreed to care for the children before contacting CWA.

The family, having made a Voluntary Request for Services, is then assigned to the Office of Field Services (OFS) Application Unit. This unit will assign the request for services to a CWA case manager. If a family member or friend has been recommended as a prospective foster parent, the OFS case manager is responsible for visiting the home, interviewing the members of the household and others knowledgeable about the family, and consulting with social service providers involved with the family to ascertain if voluntary placement is the best option. If so, and if the parent agrees, the parent is eligible for participation in the Early Permanency Planning Project. The OFS case manager will complete a preliminary assessment of the prospective relative's or friend's home, including clearance through the New York State Registry of Child Abuse and Maltreatment. If the home is suitable and the relative or friend agrees to be a foster parent, the OFS case manager will refer the family to CWA's Office of Placement Services (OPS). OPS in turn will assign the case to a voluntary child care agency for a complete home study.

If no relative or family friend is willing or able to be a foster parent, the OFS case manager, in conjunction with the social service provider, will identify prospective foster parents and consult the biological parent about introducing them to the children before placement is actually necessary.

Once the OFS case manager has determined that the family is eligible for participation in the Early Permanency Planning Project, the parent immediately signs a voluntary placement agreement, which includes an optional addendum that confirms the parent's participation in the project and describes a specific triggering event for foster care placement; in most cases, this event will be the parent's hospitalization. The parent may wish to stipulate that the children should be discharged from foster care when the parent leaves the hospital. This voluntary placement agreement remains valid for three months until a placement is located or place-

Exhibit 16-1
Information Required to Enter the Early Permanency Planning Project

Information about the parents and children
- names and birth dates of all members of the parent's household

- address and telephone number of the parent's home

- names and locations of any parents or children outside the home (including the agency, facility, and CWA case number for any child currently in foster care)

- all relevant information on parent(s) and children from collateral sources (e.g., health care providers, school officials)

- children's HIV status, if child is known to be HIV positive (disclosure must adhere to confidentiality regulations)

- time frame for placement (approximate date children will enter care, if known)

- name and telephone number of primary service provider or other referral source (e.g., Division of AIDS Services case manager, hospital social worker)

Information required only if there is a relative or family friend willing to act as a foster parent
- name and date of birth of prospective foster parent

- relationship to family (relative, godparent, friend)

- address and telephone number of prospective foster parent

- household composition of prospective foster home

- initial assessment of prospective foster parent's ability to care for the children, including discussion of the condition of the potential foster home

---

ment actually begins. Parents should be advised that they can contact a lawyer before they sign the agreement.

If the referral is for the identification of a foster home (and not to designate a relative's or friend's home), the OPS will determine which voluntary child care agency is most appropriate for the referral. Agencies participating in the Early Permanency Planning Project will specialize in particular geographical areas, to increase the likelihood of locating a foster home near the children's home and school.

If the referral is for a designated relative or a friend, the voluntary child care agency then performs a Special Home Study. If the designated home is disapproved, the OFS case manager should consult with the family to determine if there are other relatives or friends who would be willing to act as foster parents for the child or children.

Once the voluntary child care agency has found a promising foster parent, staff members will contact the OFS case manager, the social service provider (if one exists), and the family, to schedule a meeting between the family and the potential foster parent. If the initial meeting goes well and the family is able to arrange the services required by the children, the agency and the family may arrange further meetings or outings to give the children an opportunity to become familiar and comfortable with the prospective foster parent gradually.

If the voluntary child care agency decides, based on feedback from the parent(s), children, and potential foster parent, that a prospective foster parent is not a good match for the children, the agency can either search for another promising foster parent, or notify OPS that it cannot identify a foster parent for the children. The agency must notify the OPS as soon as possible. The OPS worker will contact the OFS case manager to determine when placement may be anticipated. Based on that anticipated time period, OPS may, if a placement must be found speedily, make a referral to one of the other agencies participating in the project. If enough time exists, OPS will most likely direct the initially selected agency to continue its efforts to identify an appropriate foster home.

Voluntary child care agencies receive no funding for services to Early Permanency Planning Project families until a formal foster care placement has been completed. They must absorb the costs of services they provide in advance of placement, which may include identifying and preparing a foster home, and providing counseling to the parent with AIDS and to his or her children. Once placement occurs, the agencies are reimbursed for Early Permanency Planning Project families on the same basis as for services to other foster care families, through a per diem rate set by the New York State Department of Social Services. Foster parents caring for Early Permanency Planning Project children receive a board rate established by the New York State Department of Social Services, which varies depending upon the age and needs of the child.

If the Early Permanency Planning Project family is eligible for Social Security Act Title IV-E reimbursement, or for Emergency Assistance to Families, 50 percent of the costs of service and care are funded with federal reimbursements, 25 percent by state funds, and 25 percent by the city's own tax revenues. If the family is not eligible for either federal program, then the costs of care and services are covered 50 percent by state funds and 50 percent by city tax levy funds.

Surrender of Parental Rights

After a home is identified or certified (in the case of a relative or friend's home), the OFS case manager will remain in contact with the family and, when placement becomes necessary, arrange with the voluntary child care agency to transport the children to the foster home. If adoption is the plan for the children at the time of long-term placement, the OFS case manager may present the parent with the option of surrendering parental rights at that point, in order to expedite the adoption proceedings.

Surrender of parental rights should be broached only in cases where the parent feels comfortable with adoption proceedings beginning prior to his or her death, however. Parents should be advised that they can contact a lawyer, and should be given the listing of AIDS legal services providers that is attached to the Early Permanency Planning procedures. Parents are most likely to surrender parental rights when they have developed a close relationship with the foster family and are therefore reassured that the children will continue to visit between the two homes while the parent is alive. This option may protect a parent who wants to ensure that a specific relative cannot take custody of the children at the time of death.

Emergency and Respite Care

Once a foster home is designated for the children, the foster parent can serve as a resource for short-term foster care whenever the parent is hospitalized. Often, HIV-ill parents may be hospitalized with an opportunistic infection but then recover and be able to resume caring for their children. The presence of a designated foster parent will ease a parent's anxiety about the care of his or her children by providing a caretaker who will be available on short notice. Once the parent has signed a voluntary placement agreement, the children can be placed in the foster home identified for them whenever it is necessary.

Even a parent who is not hospitalized, but who needs a respite from the stress of parenting while fighting his or her illness, can place children with CWA for as long as necessary in the foster home prepared for them. These extended visits to the prospective foster home will not only give the parent needed relief, but will also help promote a sympathetic and gradual transition for the children. At least one such overnight stay in the foster home before the long-term placement is strongly recommended.

Support Services after Placement

Agencies participating in the Early Permanency Planning Project will develop specialized services, such as support groups and bereavement counseling, for the children to help them adjust to the loss of their parents to AIDS and make the transition to a new environment.

Next Steps

As the Early Permanency Planning Project moves ahead, there are several issues to consider.

Therapeutic Services

The project will need to assist families in coping with the dying process. We plan to explore various intervention strategies to determine which are most effective in addressing this most difficult issue. The project will examine and attempt to meet the needs of the family members surviving the death of the person with AIDS, particularly the therapeutic service needs of children and foster families. We anticipate that children in these families will require individual and group interventions. Families may also require various family interventions to assist them in addressing their losses and in building a future without their loved one. Services to foster and adoptive homes may include support groups or other approaches to assisting the substitute family in assuming their role with the birth family.

Data Collection

We intend to collect data on the number of children currently entering care through the project as a result of an AIDS-related death in the family. In addition, to anticipate future needs, we will identify the growth in the use of the project's services over time.

Work Group

We will develop a work group to identify and resolve current and anticipated problems in service delivery. The initial group will consist of representatives of the four voluntary child care agencies chosen to pilot the project, and of CWA and the New York State Department of Social Services. As deemed appropriate, the work group will be enlarged to include representatives of the Human Resources Administration's Division of AIDS Services, CWA-contracted prevention programs, hospital-based social service providers, legal service providers, community-based organizations, and other groups.

Training
Training is crucial to the project. We will work closely with the pilot agencies to develop a training curriculum. The agencies will continue to use existing training resources for families and children, and CWA has developed a specialized training curriculum for field and case management personnel.

Conclusion
Permanency planning for minor children may be the most painful task a parent can face. Nevertheless, it is important for families to make custody plans before a crisis arises. The project's current experience shows that referrals are being made without sufficient lead time to ease youngsters into foster care. Of the families referred to the project, most have come in on an emergency basis. As a result, most of the parents have not been able to visit with the foster parents before their deaths. Service providers working with these families should be encouraged to explore permanency planning during the early stages of illness, rather than later.

V

FUTURE NEEDS

17

Recommendations

Carol Levine

THE DEATH OF A PARENT is a profound loss, no matter at what age it occurs or from what cause. When a parent dies, a child loses not only current care, support, and nurturing, but also a link with the past and the possibility of a shared future. Nothing can make up for that loss. A child does not "get over" the death of a parent, but he or she can get past it.

To do that, concerned family members and new guardians, professionals, and policymakers can help youngsters whose parent or parents have died of HIV/AIDS. Several authors in this volume offered recommendations for future action; see in particular Chapter 2 by Barbara Draimin and Chapter 12 by Mildred Pinott. This final chapter contains some general recommendations in the areas of service, research, education, and training.

Service

The death of a parent, in bureaucratic terms, closes a case. For the surviving children and their new guardians, however, the case may have changed but it is very much open. At present there is no system to bridge the gap between the AIDS-specific entitlements and services that benefit not only the person with AIDS but also their dependents and the entitlements and services that may be available to the new guardian and the surviving youngsters.

This gap in services is most obvious for workers and clients in the New York City Human Resources Administration's Division of AIDS Services (DAS). Some community-based agencies are beginning to provide transition services and more are needed. In addition, there is an urgent need for a more comprehensive, citywide approach. This need could be met by the creation of a transition unit at the Human Resources Administration.

A transition unit, managed by specially trained staff, would help families to set up new living arrangements and obtain benefits to which they are entitled. It would refer them to appropriate community-based legal and mental health services and bereavement counseling. Ideally, staff would have access to a flexible discretionary fund that could be used to pay for one-time special expenses associated with taking over the care of surviving children. Such expenses might be for clothing, furniture, moving, or other justifiable costs.

At present most DAS cases are closed within one to two months after the client's death. A transition unit would take over for an additional six months, with the option of extending services for a few more months in special circumstances.

Research
A second area of need is research. The gaps in knowledge are as significant as the gaps in services. Several promising areas for research are:

- epidemiological studies that link HIV-infected fathers to their children, so that estimates of the numbers of orphaned children can be more comprehensive

- long-term follow-up of surviving children and their new guardians to determine what elements appear to be significant in promoting continuity, family or sibling cohesiveness, and positive outcomes

- qualitative studies of different family coping strategies, and the role of cultural background, religious beliefs, and socioeconomic status in influencing choices about placement

- comparisons of different methods of encouraging parents to plan for the future care of their children

- research on the best ways to provide AIDS risk-reduction programs for adolescents so that teens who know at first hand the devastation of AIDS can be helped to reduce their own risky behavior

Research findings in all these areas should be used to evaluate current services and policies, modify them where necessary, and create even more sensitive and effective programs.

Information, Education, and Training

As information about the needs of surviving children and families, available resources, and research findings becomes known, it must be disseminated to the wide variety of professionals who work with youth and families. These include teachers and school administrators, judges and attorneys, workers in the many agencies involved with juvenile justice, staff at youth-serving organizations, and mental health and social work professionals. Finally, legislators and the public must be educated about the needs of vulnerable youngsters and their families, so that resources will be available to fund these efforts.

This book and the conference that inspired it are the first steps in a long journey. The road ahead may be full of obstacles, but with the lives and futures of so many young people at stake there can be no stopping and no going back.

Resource Guide

THIS GUIDE LISTS organizations that provide non-medical services to children, parents, and other family members with HIV/AIDS or affected by HIV/AIDS. Such services include mental health care, psychotherapy, and bereavement counseling; estate planning, wills, custody planning, and other legal assistance; home care, case management, benefits and entitlements assistance, and other social services. In most cases, a contact person is named in order to facilitate access to services. Because staff will change over time, however, the contact information is only a guide for initial inquiries.

This guide is intended to help family members and providers learn more about available services in New York City, but it is by no means a comprehensive listing. The New York City Department of Health publishes *Family AIDS Resource Guide*, available through the New York City AIDS Program Services' HIV Resource Library at (212) 788-4283 or through AIDS Media and Materials at (212) 285-4631. For a copy of *HIV/AIDS Resources for Adolescents*, published by the AIDS and Adolescents Network of New York, call the Network at (212) 925-6675.

Twenty hospitals in New York City are designated as AIDS Centers (see next page). They provide medical services to patients with HIV/AIDS and also provide case management and other support services. Patients at these hospitals can request assistance with family issues from the social work departments of these hospitals.

Hospitals Designated as AIDS Centers

Bronx
Bronx-Lebanon Hospital Center
Montefiore Medical Center

Brooklyn
Brookdale Hospital
Interfaith Medical Center
Lutheran Medical Center
University Hospital at SUNY Health
   Science Center

Manhattan
Beth Israel Medical Center
Cabrini Medical Center
Lenox Hill Hospital
The Mount Sinai Medical Center
The New York Hospital
North General Hospital

The Presbyterian Hospital
St. Clare's Hospital and Health
   Center
St. Luke's-Roosevelt Hospital Center
St. Vincent's Hospital and Medical
   Center of New York

Queens
The New York Hospital Medical
   Center of Queens (formerly Booth
   Memorial Medical Center)

Staten Island
Bayley Seton Hospital
St. Vincent's Medical Center of
   Richmond
Staten Island University Hospital

ACTUAL (AIDS Children Teaching Us About Love)
SUNY Health Science Center
450 Clarkson Avenue, Box 1203/Brooklyn, NY 11203
(718) 270-2598

Provides support groups and activities for biological and foster parents caring for HIV-positive children. Also sponsors HIV-positive children in summer camp.

Area served: Brooklyn
Contact: Johanna Dowdon
Fee: none

Joseph P. Addabbo Family Health Center
67-10 Rockaway Beach Boulevard/Arverne, NY 11692
(718) 945-7150, ext. 262

Offers Project HELP, a comprehensive health care services program for parents with HIV/AIDS, their children, foster parents, and new guardians. Includes a mental health clinic for individual, family, and group counseling. Also provides health case management services.

Area served: Queens (Rockaway Peninsula, Broad Channel)
Contact: Fern Zager, ACSW (718) 945-7150 ext. 262; Jamila Ali, HIV Nurse
Coordinator (718) 945-7150 ext. 246
Fee: sliding scale based on income and family size for patients without coverage;
Medicaid, Medicare, and private insurance accepted for all other patients

Advocates for Children of New York
24-16 Bridge Plaza South/Long Island City, NY 11101
(718) 729-8866

Serves parents with HIV/AIDS, their children, children with HIV/AIDS, foster parents, new guardians, and other affected family members. Provides educational advocacy around the needs of school children with HIV/AIDS and school children from families with HIV/AIDS. Will also provide group trainings on educational rights. Spanish available.

Area served: New York City
Contact: callers seeking assistance for individual cases should request an intake worker; callers for group training should ask for Vivian Brady
Fee: none

AIDS Center of Queens County
97-45 Queens Boulevard, Suite 1220/Rego Park, NY 11374
(718) 896-2500
or
175-61 Hillside Avenue, 4th Floor/Jamaica, NY 11432
(718) 739-2500

Serves parents with AIDS, their children, and other affected family members by providing individual, group, and family therapy and bereavement counseling. Provides assistance in custody and estate planning. Also provides social case management and benefits/entitlements assistance. Spanish available.

Area served: Queens
Contact: to enroll as a client at either office, call for an intake appointment; if calling the Rego Park office, ask for Jim Wilson
Fee: none

AIDS Resource Center
275 7th Avenue, 12th Floor/New York, NY 10001
(212) 633-2500

Serves parents with AIDS and their minor children. Provides housing, case management services, mental health services, and an activities program to all clients. *Clients must be referred through the New York City Division of AIDS Services Housing Unit.* Spanish available.

Area served: New York City
Contact: Division of AIDS Services at (212) 645-7070; ask for the Housing Unit
Fee: apartment fee consists of 25 percent of SSI entitlements; all other services free

All-Craft Center
25 St. Mark's Place, 2nd Floor/New York, NY 10003
(212) 260-3650

Serves mostly homeless population. Provides self-help meetings based on a
Narcotics Anonymous model. Also offers an "HIV-positive Anonymous" group,
programs for adolescents whose parents are chemically dependent, and programs
for adolescents who have a history of substance abuse. Staffed by only a few
professionally trained volunteers.

Area served: New York City
Contact: Intake Office
Fee: none

American Red Cross in Greater New York
150 Amsterdam Avenue/New York, NY 10023
(212) 875-2194

Provides transportation services to parents with HIV/AIDS, their children, foster
parents, and new guardians. Spanish available.

Area served: New York City
Contact: Barbara Reisman
Fee: none

Babies Hospital
Special Needs Clinic
Columbia Presbyterian Medical Center
622 West 168th Street, Room 619N/New York, NY 10032
(212) 305-3093

Provides bereavement and group, family, and individual therapy to parents with
HIV/AIDS, their children (up to age 18), foster parents, new guardians, and
affected siblings. Also provides client evaluation, psychopharmacology, and
parent training. Spanish available.

Area served: Bronx, Manhattan
Contact: Sheila Ryan, MSW
Fee: sliding scale; Medicaid accepted

Beth Israel Medical Center
Well Children in AIDS Families Project
1st Avenue and East 16th Street/New York, NY 10003
(212) 420-2851

Provides mental health services to uninfected children (ages 5–20) of parents with AIDS, including short-term and ongoing therapy, family treatment, group work and bereavement counseling. Also assists with custody and placement issues through advocacy and referral.

Area served: New York City and surrounding areas
Contact: Lockhart McKelvy, CSW
Fee: Medicaid accepted for group services; no fee for other services

Herbert G. Birch Residential Children's Center
594 East 53rd Street/Brooklyn, NY 11203
(718) 528-5754

Provides a residence for disabled children and children with AIDS. Also runs a one-week summer camp for children with AIDS and their infected or affected family members.

Area served: New York City Area
Contact: Executive Office
Fee: none

Body Positive
2095 Broadway, Suite 306/New York, NY 10023
(212) 721-1618

Offers support groups to parents and children with HIV/AIDS and their affected family members, including siblings, friends, and lovers. Also offers educational forums on living with HIV/AIDS and disease management. Spanish available.

Area served: Bronx, Brooklyn, Manhattan, Queens
Contact: Carmen Navarro (Education and Outreach) or Michelle Serracco (Director of Support Services)
Fee: none

Bronx AIDS Services
1 Fordham Plaza, Suite 903/Bronx, NY 10458
(718) 295-5605

Serves parents with HIV/AIDS and affected family members, especially adolescents. Offers an adolescent support group, social case management services, and legal services. Spanish available.

Area served: Bronx
Contact: Isa Mariella Martinez, CSW
Fee: none

Bronx-Lebanon Hospital
Family Outreach Program
Department of Social Services
1650 Selwyn Avenue, 7C/Bronx, NY 10459
(718) 960-1068 or 960-1060

Serves parents with AIDS, their uninfected children (up to age 21), foster parents, new guardians, and other affected family members. Provides bereavement counseling; group, individual and family therapy; support groups for teens and new guardians; assistance with guardianship and custody planning; benefits and entitlements assistance; and assistance in arranging child care during hospitalization of a parent. Spanish available.

Area served: Bronx; accepts referrals from other boroughs on a per case basis
Contact: Rudene Scipio
Fee: none

Bronx Municipal Hospital Day Care Center
Pelham Parkway South and Eastchester Road, Van Etten 6B/Bronx, NY 10461
(718) 918-4535

Offers a day care program for children with HIV/AIDS ages 2–7.

Area served: Bronx
Contact: Carolyn Lelyveld
Fee: none

Brooklyn AIDS Task Force
465 Dean Street/Brooklyn, NY 11217
(718) 783-0883, ext. 22

Provides case management services to parents and children with HIV/AIDS and their affected family members. Gives referrals for mental health services, legal services, and home care. Spanish, French, and Creole available.

Area served: Brooklyn
Contact: Vincenta Cintron-Perez, Case Manager
Fee: none

Brooklyn Center for Families in Crisis
535 East 17th Street/Brooklyn, NY 11226
(718) 282-0010

Provides bereavement counseling and psychotherapy to parents with HIV/AIDS, their children (both HIV-infected and uninfected), foster parents, new guardians, and other affected family members.

Area served: Brooklyn
Contact: Jennifer Hall, CSW, Intake Coordinator
Fee: patient fee $65; Medicaid, Medicare, private insurance accepted

Brooklyn Legal Services
HIV Project
105 Court Street/Brooklyn, NY 11201
(718) 237-5546

Provides legal services to parents with AIDS, their children, foster parents, new guardians, and other affected family members. Services include wills/estate planning and custody planning. Also provides services around other legal issues such as entitlements, foster care, access to health care, and housing. Spanish available.

Area served: Brooklyn
Contact: Lauren Shapiro
Fee: none (provides services to low-income individuals only)

Brookwood Child Care
25 Washington Street/Brooklyn, NY 11201
(718) 596-5555, ext. 530

Provides a broad range of services to parents with AIDS, their HIV-infected and uninfected children, foster parents, new guardians, and other family members. Offers adoption services, a foster care program, two group homes for adolescents, a preventive service program, and a family day care program. Services provided within these programs include mental health services, respite care, case management, and legal services (for families within the foster care program). Spanish and Haitian available.

Area served: Brooklyn
Contact: Marilyn Barney
Fee: none

Camp Good Days and Special Times
1332 Pittsford Mendon Road/Mendon, NY 14506
(716) 624-5555 or (716) 427-2650

Summer camp in Branchport, NY, for children who have a parent or sibling with AIDS, or who have lost a parent or sibling to AIDS.

Area served: New York City area
Contact: Annie Pixley
Fee: $25 registration fee; scholarships based on need

Caribbean Women's Health Association
2725 Church Avenue/Brooklyn, NY 11226
(718) 826-2942

Serves parents with AIDS and their affected family members. Provides individual and group counseling and social and health case management services. Spanish, French, and Creole available.

Area served: New York City
Contact: Dr. Ady Turnier or Anibal Cordero
Fee: none

Center for Children and Families (Safe Space)
133 West 46th Street/New York, NY 10036
(212) 354-7233

Serves HIV-infected and uninfected adolescents (ages 13–22). Offers intensive and comprehensive case management services. Also offers mental health services (including bereavement counseling), legal referrals, and a residence for 12 adolescents with HIV (opening September 1993). Spanish available.

Area served: New York City area
Contact: Director, Mental Health Clinic, or the HIV and Health Coordinator
Fee: sliding scale and Medicaid accepted for mental health services; no fees for other services

Child Welfare Administration
(see New York City Human Resources Administration)

Children's Aid Society
Preventive Service Program
350 East 88th Street, 2nd Floor/New York, NY 10128
(212) 876-9715

Serves parents with HIV/AIDS and their children (up to age 18), who are eligible for preventive services under CWA guidelines (i.e., one or more children in the home must be at risk for foster care placement). Offers social case management, homemaking services (arranged through CWA only), and referrals for mental health and legal services. Spanish available.

Area served: upper Manhattan (north of 96th Street, community districts 9, 10, 11, 12)
Contact: Geraldine Cossen
Fee: none

Children's Hope Foundation
295 Lafayette Street, Suite 801/New York, NY 10012
(212) 941-7432

Serves children with HIV/AIDS (up to age 13). Provides activities, hospital emergency funds, child care necessities, and treatment and transportation assistance.

Area served: New York City; Newark, NJ
Contact: Sofia Mortada or Stacey Rouse
Fee: none

Church Avenue Merchants Block Association (CAMBA)
1720 Church Avenue, 2nd Floor/Brooklyn, NY 11226
(718) 287-0010

Provides social case management services and mental health services to parents with HIV/AIDS and their uninfected children, ages 7–18. Also provides bereavement services to any family members who have lost a loved one to AIDS. Haitian and Spanish available.

Area served: Brooklyn
Contact: Paula Smith
Fee: none

Community Counseling and Mediation
50 Court Street, Suite 601/Brooklyn, NY 11201
(718) 802-0666

Provides counseling, preventive services, outreach, and education to foster parents.

Area served: Brooklyn, Manhattan, Staten Island
Contact: Marjorie Saldivar
Fee: based on sliding scale; Medicaid, Medicare, private insurance accepted

Department of Health
(see New York City Department of Health)

Discipleship Outreach Ministries
5711 4th Avenue/Brooklyn, NY 11220
(718) 492-4436

Serves parents with HIV/AIDS and their children with HIV/AIDS. Also serves foster parents, new guardians, and other affected family members. Provides social case management, advocacy, other supportive services and referrals.

Area served: Brooklyn
Contact: Sara Gonzalez
Fee: Medicaid accepted for case management services; all other supportive and educational services free

Division of AIDS Services
(see New York City Human Resources Administration)

Dominican Sisters Family Health Services
279 Alexander Avenue/Bronx, NY 10454
(718) 665-6557

Serves parents with HIV/AIDS, their infected and uninfected children, foster parents, new guardians, and other affected family members. Provides bereavement services and psychotherapy (group, family, and individual); personal care attendants, housekeeping services, and nursing care; social and health case management; and a mothers' socialization group and therapeutic playroom. Some Spanish available.

Area served: Bronx (Mott Haven)
Contact: callers should phone between 8:30 AM and 4:30 PM, Monday through Friday
Fee: Medicaid and third-party reimbursements accepted; free services provided where appropriate or until entitlements are secured

The Door
121 Avenue of the Americas, 3rd Floor/New York, NY 10013
(212) 941-9090

Serves HIV-positive and HIV-negative adolescents (ages 12–21) from families with HIV/AIDS. Also serves affected adolescent family members (siblings, nieces, nephews). Provides bereavement counseling and psychotherapy; wills and estate planning; custody planning; and social and health case management. Spanish available.

Area served: New York City
Contact: Sylvia Muniz for HIV services; Jill Chaifetz for legal services
Fee: none

Early Permanency Planning Project
(see New York City Human Resources Administration)

Family Dynamics
154 Christopher Street, 2nd Floor/New York, NY 10014
(212) 255-8484

Serves parents with HIV/AIDS, their children (up to age 18), new guardians, and kinship parents. Provides a variety of preventive services including case management, counseling, family outings, and parenting skills. The "High-Risk" Families program is aimed at providing a broad range of services to families with HIV/AIDS and/or substance abuse. The Foster Care Discharge program works with families whose children are in foster care, toward the goal of reuniting the whole family. The Grandparents in Action Project (GAP) provides support to grandparents who have taken on primary parenting responsibilities. Spanish available.

Area served: Brooklyn, Manhattan
Contact: Marlienne Christian, Program Director (718) 783-6666; Herve Bertrand, Program Director (718) 455-2300; Crystal George, Program Director (212) 255-8484
Fee: none

Gay Men's Health Crisis
129 West 20th Street/New York, NY 10011
(212) 337-3620 (for general intake)
(212) 337-3504 (for legal department)

Large AIDS service agency that serves parents with HIV/AIDS, their infected and uninfected children, other extended family members, new guardians, and foster parents. Provides a broad variety of social services including home care, case management, and pediatric buddy services. Also offers a full range of legal services including immigration, landlord/tenant, insurance, discrimination, and debtor/creditor. Will also assist individuals to become legal guardians. Spanish available.

Area served: New York City
Contact: legal department—(212) 337-3504; other services—call the Intake Unit of Client Services on Mondays after 10:00 AM at (212) 337-3620
Fee: none

God's Love We Deliver
895 Amsterdam Avenue/New York, NY 10025
(212) 865-6500 (for meal delivery)
(212) 865-4900 (for nutrition education)

Provides meal delivery to homebound people with AIDS and their dependent children up to 18 years old. Also provides nutrition counseling and education to all people with HIV/AIDS. Spanish and some French available.

Area served: New York City and parts of Hudson County, NJ
Contact: meal delivery—(212) 865-6500; nutrition education—(212) 865-4900
Fee: none

Greenwich House
AIDS Mental Health Project
80 Fifth Avenue, 10th Floor/New York, NY 10011
(212) 691-2900

Provides parents with HIV/AIDS and their affected family members with group, family, and individual counseling, including bereavement issues.

Area served: New York City, Long Island, New Jersey
Contact: Michele Fontaine
Fee: sliding scale; Medicaid accepted

Hamilton-Madison House
Teen Outreach Project
50 Madison Street/New York, NY 10038
(212) 732-4705

Provides group, family, and individual psychotherapy and bereavement counseling to all family members affected by or living with HIV/AIDS. Children must be between 12 and 22 years old. Spanish, Cantonese, and Mandarin available.

Area served: Manhattan
Contact: Gwen Tarack
Fee: sliding scale; Medicaid accepted

Harlem Dowling Westside Children and Family Center
2096 7th Avenue/New York, NY 10027
(212) 749-3656

Serves parents with HIV/AIDS, their infected and uninfected children, foster parents, new guardians, and other affected family members. Provides mental health services, social case management services, and parent aides for home care assistance. Also provides primary medical care, foster care, adoption, and preventive services. AIDS-specific programs include the Women's Initiative Program for women with HIV/AIDS and an early custody planning program for parents with HIV/AIDS. Spanish available.

Area served: Harlem and the Upper West Side of Manhattan; an additional foster care office is located in Queens
Contact: follow recorded instructions
Fee: none

Harlem Interfaith Counseling Service
Community Consultation and Education Unit
215 West 125th Street/New York, NY 10027
(212) 662-8613

Provides services to HIV-affected children, youth, and new guardians. Includes mental health, bereavement counseling, and other support services.

Area served: upper Manhattan
Contact: Doris Dennard or Vanessa Marshall
Fee: none

Henry Street Settlement
Community Consultation Center
40 Montgomery Street/New York, NY 10002
(212) 233-5032

Serves parents with HIV/AIDS, their uninfected children, foster parents, new guardians. Provides individual, group, and family bereavement counseling and psychotherapy. Also provides school-based bereavement support group for healthy children whose parents have died or are dying of AIDS. Works to provide orphans with extended families with physical and psychological well being. Will assist with kinship placement of children. Provides social and health case management. Spanish, French, Hindi, German, and three dialects of Chinese available.

Area served: primarily lower Manhattan and the Lower East Side
Contact: Lela Charney, Director of HIV Services
Fee: sliding scale; Medicaid, Medicare, and third-party insurance accepted

Hetrick-Martin Institute

401 West Street/New York, NY 10014
(212) 633-8920

Provides adolescents with HIV/AIDS (ages 12–21) and their affected family members with group, family, and individual counseling. Also provides adolescents with support groups, social and health case management, peer education, youth internships, socialization, and food clothing and GED classes for homeless youth. Spanish and Creole available.

Area served: New York City
Contact: George Ayala, Director of Client Services
Fee: none

HIV Law Project

80 Fifth Avenue/New York, NY 10011
(212) 645-8863

Provides legal advice and/or representation to low-income parents with HIV/AIDS and new guardians. Covers a broad range of issues including custody and guardianship, wills and estate planning, housing, public benefits, health care, child support, divorce, health care proxy, and power of attorney. Spanish available.

Area served: Manhattan
Contact: Cynthia Reed
Fee: none

Hospital Audiences, Inc.

220 West 42nd Street, 13th Floor/New York, NY 10036
(212) 575-7681

Provides parents with HIV/AIDS and adolescents with mental health services, education and prevention, and in-hospital and in-school performances. Spanish available for education program.

Area served: New York City
Contact: Patty Reitkopf
Fee: none

Housing Works
594 Broadway, Suite 700/New York, NY 10012
(212) 966-0466

Provides scatter-site housing and intensive supportive services to parents with
HIV/AIDS and their children who are homeless or at risk of homelessness. Also
provides a job training program, a harm reduction center (for chemically
dependent people), a needle exchange program, mental health referrals, peer
support, and recreational and nutritional services. Spanish available.

Area served: Bronx, Brooklyn, Manhattan
Contact: ask for the intake program
Fee: none

Informed School Project
(see SUNY Health Science Center)

Jewish Board of Family and Children's Services (JBFCS)
120 West 57th Street/New York, NY 10025
See phone numbers below

The AIDS Services Program provides mental health and bereavement counseling,
social case management, scattered-site supportive housing, day treatment, and
volunteer friendly visitors to parents with HIV/AIDS, their infected and
uninfected children, foster parents, new guardians, and other affected family
members. Spanish, Russian, and Hebrew available.

Area served: New York City
Contact: Bronx—Helen Mullin, CSW (718) 931-2600; Brooklyn—Adina
Shapiro, CSW (718) 855-6900; Manhattan—Toni Mufson, CSW (212) 632-
4695; Staten Island—Janice Gross, CSW (718) 761-9800
Fee: sliding scale

Rose F. Kennedy Center
Children Evaluation and Rehabilitation Center (CERC)
1410 Pelham Parkway South/Bronx, NY 10461
(718) 430-3972

Serves HIV-infected and uninfected children (up to age 21) of parents with HIV/
AIDS and any family member caring for a child with HIV-infection. Provides
bereavement counseling; group, family, and individual therapy; support groups
for Spanish-speaking care givers; social and health case management; referral
services; and developmental and educational services. Limited counseling in
Spanish available.

Area served: New York City and suburbs
Contact: Anna Alejandro
Fee: sliding scale; Medicaid and private insurance accepted

Lakeside Family and Children's Services
185 Montague Street/Brooklyn, NY 11201
(718) 237-9700

Provides mental health services, case management services, and foster care
placement for children of parents with HIV/AIDS (or who have died of HIV/
AIDS) and foster parents.

Area served: New York City
Contact: Jan Goldberg
Fee: none

Leake and Watts Children's Home
487 South Broadway, Suite 201/Yonkers, NY 10705
(914) 376-4415
Specialized Foster Care Helpline: (914) 423-5273

Provides foster care services to both HIV-infected and uninfected children (up to
age 18). Provides other services to parents with HIV/AIDS, foster parents and
kinship foster parents. These include support groups, bereavement counseling,
referrals for home care services, social and health case management. Also
distributes a quarterly newsletter. Spanish available.

Area served: Brooklyn, Bronx, Manhattan, Westchester County
Contact: Kathy Goodbody, Director of State Training Grant (914) 376-4415
Fee: none

Legal Aid Society
Community Law Offices
230 East 106th Street/New York, NY 10029
(212) 722-2000

Serves parents with HIV/AIDS, new guardians, and other affected family members. Includes issues around standby guardianship, entitlements, and landlord/tenant.

Area served: Bronx, Manhattan, Queens, and patients at the following hospitals: Beth Israel, Metropolitan, Mount Sinai, North Central Bronx, Montefiore, and Bronx-Lebanon
Contact: Diane La Gamma, Esq., and Elizabeth A. Hay, Esq.
Fee: none

Legal Aid Society
Juvenile Rights Division
15 Park Row/New York, NY 10038
(212) 613-3890

Provides legal representation to HIV-infected and uninfected children of parents with HIV/AIDS. Covers Family Court proceedings, neglect, abuse, delinquency, and termination of parental rights. (For delinquency cases, the agency represents children up to 16 years old; for neglect and abuse cases, the agency represents children up to 18 years old.) Language interpreters available.

Area served: New York City
Contact: Nanette Schrandt, Director, Juvenile Services Unit
Fee: none

Lower East Side Family Union
84 Stanton Street, 3rd Floor/New York, NY 10002
(212) 260-0040

Provides parents with HIV/AIDS and their children with bereavement and other mental health counseling, custody planning, personal care attendants, house-keeping services, and social case management. Also provides a women's support group and referrals. Spanish and Chinese available.

Area served: Manhattan (Lower East Side)
Contact: Ericka Deglau
Fee: none

Mayer-Avedon Women's Support Groups
7 East 14th Street/New York, NY 10003
(212) 989-6649

Provides services to uninfected family members of an HIV-infected person, such as wives, long-term partners, parents and grandparents of an infected child, and uninfected children (ages 4–11) of parents with HIV/AIDS. Offers support groups for uninfected wives or partners of men with HIV/AIDS. Will soon offer a support group for uninfected children. Some Spanish available.

Area served: New York City
Contact: leave message at above number
Fee: sliding scale based on income

Minority Task Force on AIDS
505 8th Avenue, 16th Floor/New York, NY 10018
See phone numbers below

Serves parents with HIV/AIDS and their children. Provides support groups, wills and estate planning, custody planning, entitlements assistance, discrimination advocacy, social case management, home visits, meal programs, education, a clothing bank, and a residence with a management program. Spanish available.

Area served: New York City (emphasis on upper Manhattan)
Contact: Client Services Department—Pat Jerido (212) 864-4046; Housing Department—Richard Skinner (212) 927-5161; Education Department—Mark Carter (212) 563-8340
Fee: none

Montefiore Medical Center
Adolescent AIDS Program
111 East 210th Street/Bronx, NY 10467
(718) 882-0023 or (718) 920-2129

Provides comprehensive medical, psychological, and case-management services to adolescents with HIV/AIDS, ages 13–21. Will refer affected family members to an appropriate service program. Spanish available.

Area served: New York City (emphasis on Bronx)
Contact: Miriam Ramos or Colleen Jones
Fee: sliding scale; private insurance and Medicaid accepted; free initial consultation can be arranged

New Alternatives for Children
37 West 26th Street/New York, NY 10010
(212) 696-1550

Provides comprehensive support services to hospitalized boarder children (up to 18 years old) and their families (including parents with HIV/AIDS, siblings, and foster parents). Provides individual and family counseling, bereavement counseling, support groups, medical services, respite care, transportation, children's and sibling groups, social and health case management, and referrals. The prevention, foster care and adoption programs help children leave the hospital and live in the community. Spanish available.

Area served: New York City
Contact: Susan Schechter
Fee: none

New York City Department of Health
Bureau for Families with Special Needs
111 Livingston Street, Room 2022/New York, NY 11201
(718) 643-7337 or (718) 643-7630

Offers resources and information about other services for families living with HIV/AIDS.

Area served: New York City
Contact: Karen Hopkins, MD (718) 643-7337; Colin Brown (718) 643-7630
Fee: none

New York City Human Resources Administration
Child Welfare Administration
80 Lafayette Street/New York, NY 10013

For families seeking foster care placement for their children, homemaking and housekeeping, adoption services, preventive services and family preservation services, please call the numbers below. The office that provides services is based on the Community District in which the applicant lives.

Area served: New York City
Contact: Bronx—(718) 716-0550 or (718) 579-8890; Brooklyn—(718) 522-8209, (718) 826-5500, or (718) 348-8015; Manhattan—(212) 266-2687 or (212) 614-7037; Queens—(718) 481-5760; Staten Island—(718) 720-2817
Fee: none

New York City Human Resources Administration
Division of AIDS Services
241 Church Street/New York, NY 10013
(212) 645-7070

Serves Medicaid-eligible parents and children with AIDS or advanced HIV illness. Provides comprehensive services around mental health, legal issues, home care, case management, meals, housing, advocacy, burial arrangements, and other areas.

Area served: New York City
Contact: call the AIDS Serviceline, (212) 645-7070, Monday through Friday, 8:30 AM to 6:00 PM
Fee: Medicaid accepted

New York City Public Schools
Division of Student Support Services
110 Livingston Street, Room 510/Brooklyn, NY 11201
(718) 935-4042

Serves both infected and uninfected children of parents with HIV/AIDS, and any children who are at risk of dropping out of school. Support services and counseling are accessed through school guidance counselors. Other languages available.

Area served: New York City
Contact: School guidance counselor
Fee: none

New York Council on Adoptable Children
666 Broadway, Suite 820/New York, NY 10012
(212) 475-0222

Recruits prospective adoptive or custodial parents for to-be-orphaned, uninfected children who have no other family resource. Assists parents with HIV/AIDS, their uninfected children, and new guardians with custody planning. Also provides assistance with wills and estate planning.

Area served: New York City; prospective new guardians may reside almost anywhere in the nation
Contact: Algernon Thomas, MSW, Program Director
Fee: none

New York Foundling Hospital
Project Hope
1029 East 163rd Street/Bronx, NY 10459
(718) 328-9883

Provides foster care services to children with HIV/AIDS (from birth to teenage years, but primarily infants and toddlers). Also serves foster parents, kinship care guardians, standby guardians, and any other family members (including parents) who are involved in service planning for children. Offers bereavement and pastoral counseling, individual and family therapy, support groups, psychological/developmental assessments, custody planning, adoption, in-home personal care attendants, respite care, crisis intervention, social and health case management, and other programs. Spanish available.

Area served: New York City, Long Island, Westchester County
Contact: Ann Marie Rakovic, Director; foster care services accessed through CWA referrals only
Fee: none

Planned Parenthood
The Hub
349 East 149th Street, Suite 609/Bronx, NY 10451
(718) 585-5001

Provides bereavement counseling, individual counseling and psychotherapy, and social case management to parents with HIV/AIDS, their uninfected children (7 years of age and older), foster parents, new guardians, and other affected family members. Spanish available.

Area served: Bronx, Queens, upper Manhattan
Contact: Donna Bersch
Fee: none

Puerto Rican Association for Community Affairs (PRACA)
853 Broadway, 5th Floor/New York, NY 10003
(212) 673-7322

Serves parents with HIV/AIDS, their children, foster parents, and other affected family members. Provides bereavement and individual counseling, adoption planning, social and health case management, and advocacy. Spanish available.

Area served: New York City
Contact: Gilberto Cintron
Fee: none

St. Clare's Hospital and Health Center
Spellman Center for HIV-Related Disease
415 West 51st Street/New York, NY 10019
See phone numbers below

Serves parents with HIV/AIDS and their HIV-infected children. Also serves all affected family members including foster parents and new guardians. Provides a comprehensive health and mental health team in an outpatient setting. Includes mental health care, primary health care, legal assistance, a methadone program, social and health case management. Spanish available.

Area served: Greater New York Metropolitan area
Contact: Medical—(212) 459-8130; Case Management—(212) 459-8445; Dental—(212) 459-8327; Outreach—(212) 459-8406; Volunteers—(212) 459-8433
Fee: Medicaid, Medicare, and private insurance accepted; HMOs often not accepted

St. Vincent's Hospital
Supportive Care Program
153 West 11th Street/New York, NY 10011
(212) 790-7508

Provides bereavement groups for children and parents. Some Spanish available.

Area served: New York City
Contact: Kathleen Perry
Fee: none

St. Vincent's Services
Positive Caring Program
66 Boerum Place/Brooklyn, NY 11201
(718) 875-2480 or (718) 522-3700

Private foster care agency with specialized foster care for HIV-positive children. Serves HIV-infected and uninfected children, parents with HIV/AIDS, and foster parents. Provides support groups for foster and adoptive parents, bereavement counseling, psychotherapy, in-home personal care attendants, and social and health case management.

Area served: primarily Brooklyn and Queens; also Manhattan, Bronx, and Long Island
Contact: Sister Elizabeth Mullane (718) 875-2480
Fee: none

Selfhelp Community Services
440 9th Avenue/New York, NY 10001
(212) 971-5480

The New Guardian Program provides home care services, social case management, advocacy, and support services to new guardians of AIDS orphans. Assists in beginning guardianship proceedings and transferring entitlement benefits. Also provides services to parents with HIV/AIDS and their children. Spanish available.

Area served: Bronx, Brooklyn, Manhattan, Queens
Contact: Andres Campos
Fee: none

Settlement Health and Medical Services
HELP Program
314 East 104th Street/New York, NY 10029
(212) 860-0401 for case management services
(212) 410-5741 for other services

Serves parents with HIV/AIDS, their HIV-infected children (up to 2 years old), their uninfected children (up to 16 years old), and any other affected family members. Provides primary health care, individual counseling, part-time psychiatric referrals, HIV support groups for women and men, and social case management. Spanish and French available.

Area served: Bronx, Brooklyn, Manhattan, Queens
Contact: Janet Bird, for case management services
Fee: Medicaid and private insurance accepted for medical care and HIV testing; no fees for other services

Society for Seamen's Children
25 Hyatt Street/Staten Island, NY 10301
(718) 447-7740

Provides mental health services, education, custody planning, and social case management to parents with HIV/AIDS, their HIV-infected children (ages 1–11) and uninfected children (ages 0–21), foster parents, and new guardians. Some Spanish available.

Area served: Brooklyn, Manhattan, Queens, Staten Island
Contact: Lynn Kavalec, Lina Steiner
Fee: none

Spence-Chapin
Intensive Services to Families
6 East 94th Street/New York, NY 10128-0698
(212) 369-0300

Serves parents with HIV/AIDS, their infected and uninfected children (under 18 years old), and new guardians. Also provides services to affected household or significant family members. Provides adoption services, mental health services, home care services (through CWA referrals only), and social and health case management services. Money for public transportation provided to needy clients. Spanish and French available.

Area served: Manhattan Community Districts 8 and 11
Contact: Margaret Fluhr
Fee: none

SUNY Health Science Center
Infant and Child Learning Center Informed School Project
450 Clarkson Avenue, Box 1203/Brooklyn, NY 11203
(718) 270-2598

Serves children with HIV, as well as children with developmental delays. Assists parents to disclose their child's HIV status to teachers and other school personnel. Child advocates counsel and support parents as they consider their disclosure options. Provides advocacy, training, and support groups for teachers working with HIV-infected children.

Area served: New York City
Contact: Joan Hittelman, PhD
Fee: sliding scale

Upper Manhattan Task Force on AIDS
55 West 125th Street/New York, NY 10027
(212) 870-8152

Provides custody planning, estate planning, and intensive social case management to parents with HIV/AIDS, their children, foster parents, new guardians, and affected family members. Spanish available.

Area served: upper Manhattan
Contact: Carla Ford, Director, Support Services
Fee: none

Visiting Nurse Services Home Care
974-8 Morris Park Avenue
Bronx, NY 10462-3714
(212) 714-9250

Provides parents and children with HIV/AIDS with home care visits by registered nurses and home health aides. Includes social service support to affected children. Offers recreation, a support group, and individual counseling as part of a program for well adolescents (ages 8–15) who have parents with HIV/AIDS (for Bronx residents only). Also provides a Ryan White Program for children, which provides bereavement and psychosocial services (for Bronx residents only). Spanish available.

Area served: Bronx, Brooklyn, Manhattan, Queens (well adolescents program and Ryan White program for Bronx residents only)
Contact: Admissions Office, (212) 714-9250
Fee: third-party insurance including HIP, Medicaid, and Medicare; sliding-scale or free services can be arranged

Volunteers of Legal Service
17 Varick Street/New York, NY 10013-2476
(212) 966-4400

Serves parents with HIV/AIDS who are referred by hospital social workers and Division of AIDS Services caseworkers. Provides assistance with wills and estate planning, custody planning, living wills, health care proxies, and powers of attorney.

Area served: Brooklyn, Manhattan, Queens
Contact: Sara Effron, Assistant Director
Fee: none

Well Children in AIDS Families Project
(see Beth Israel Medical Center)

Women and AIDS Resource Network (WARN)
30 3rd Avenue, Suite 212/Brooklyn, NY 11217
(718) 596-6007

Provides any HIV-infected female client (adult or child) and her immediate family members with social and health case management, support groups, individual counseling, and referrals. Creole, French, and Spanish available.

Area served: New York City
Contact: Yvonne Chambers
Fee: none

Youth Advocacy Center, Inc.
55 West 14th Street, 20G/New York, NY 10013
(212) 463-7239

Provides advocacy and support services to children in foster care. Offers a
children's rights workshop and foster care rights and awareness workshop.

Area served: New York City
Contact: Betsy Krebs, Executive Director
Fee: none

Geographic Index

New York City (five boroughs)
Advocates for Children of New York
AIDS Resource Center
American Red Cross in Greater New York
Beth Israel Medical Center Well Children in AIDS Families Project
Herbert G. Birch Residential Children's Center
Camp Good Days and Special Times
Caribbean Women's Health Association
Center for Children and Families (Safe Space)
Children's Hope Foundation
The Door
Gay Men's Health Crisis
God's Love We Deliver
Greenwich House AIDS Mental Health Project
Hetrick-Martin Institute
HIV Law Project
Hospital Audiences, Inc.
Jewish Board of Family and Children's Services
Rose F. Kennedy Center CERC
Lakeside Family and Children's Services
Legal Aid Society Juvenile Rights Division
Mayer-Avedon Women's Support Groups
Minority Task Force on AIDS
Montefiore Medical Center Adolescent AIDS Program
New Alternatives for Children
NYC Department of Health Bureau for Families with Special Needs
NYC Human Resources Administration Child Welfare Administration
NYC Human Resources Administration Division of AIDS Services
NYC Public Schools Division of Student Support Services
New York Council on Adoptable Children
New York Foundling Hospital Project Hope

Puerto Rican Association for Community Affairs
St. Clare's Hospital and Health Center Spellman Center for HIV-Related Disease
St. Vincent's Hospital Supportive Care Program
SUNY Health Science Center Infant and Child Learning Center Informed
  School Project
Women and AIDS Resource Network
Youth Advocacy Center, Inc.

*Bronx**
Babies Hospital Special Needs Clinic
Body Positive
Bronx AIDS Services
Bronx-Lebanon Hospital Family Outreach Program
Bronx Municipal Hospital Day Care Center
Dominican Sisters Family Health Services
Housing Works
Leake and Watts Children's Home
Legal Aid Society Community Law Offices
Montefiore Medical Center Adolescent AIDS Program
Planned Parenthood/The Hub
St. Vincent's Services Positive Caring Program
Selfhelp Community Services
Settlement Health and Medical Services HELP Program
Visiting Nurse Services Home Care

*Brooklyn**
ACTUAL
Body Positive
Brooklyn AIDS Task Force
Brooklyn Center for Families in Crisis
Brooklyn Legal Services HIV Project
Brookwood Child Care
Church Avenue Merchants Block Association
Community Counseling and Mediation
Discipleship Outreach Ministries
Family Dynamics
Housing Works
Leake and Watts Children's Home
St. Vincent's Services Positive Caring Program
Selfhelp Community Services
Settlement Health and Medical Services HELP Program

---

*See also New York City (five boroughs).

Society for Seamen's Children
Visiting Nurse Services Home Care
Volunteers of Legal Service

Manhattan*
Babies Hospital Special Needs Clinic
Body Positive
Children's Aid Society Preventive Service Program
Community Counseling and Mediation
Family Dynamics
Hamilton-Madison House Teen Outreach Project
Harlem Dowling Westside Children and Family Center
Harlem Interfaith Counseling Service Community Consultation and
  Education Unit
Henry Street Settlement Community Consultation Center
Housing Works
Leake and Watts Children's Home
Legal Aid Society Community Law Offices
Lower East Side Family Union
Minority Task Force on AIDS
Planned Parenthood/The Hub
St. Vincent's Services Positive Caring Program
Selfhelp Community Services
Settlement Health and Medical Services HELP Program
Society for Seamen's Children
Spence-Chapin Intensive Services to Families
Upper Manhattan Task Force on AIDS
Visiting Nurse Services Home Care
Volunteers of Legal Service

Queens*
Joseph P. Addabbo Family Health Center
AIDS Center of Queens County
Body Positive
Harlem Dowling Westside Children and Family Center
Legal Aid Society Community Law Offices
Planned Parenthood/The Hub
St. Vincent's Services Positive Caring Program
Selfhelp Community Services
Settlement Health and Medical Services HELP Program
Society for Seamen's Children

---

*See also New York City (five boroughs).

Visiting Nurse Services Home Care
Volunteers of Legal Service

Staten Island*
Community Counseling and Mediation
Society for Seamen's Children

New York City Metropolitan Area
Beth Israel Medical Center Children in AIDS Families
Camp Good Days and Special Times
Center for Children and Families (Safe Space)
Rose F. Kennedy Center CERC
St. Clare's Hospital and Health Center for HIV-Related Disease

Long Island
Greenwich House AIDS Mental Health Project
New York Foundling Hospital Project Hope
St. Vincent's Services Positive Caring Program

Westchester County
Leake and Watts Children's Home
New York Foundling Hospital Project Hope

New Jersey
Children's Hope Foundation
God's Love We Deliver
Greenwich House AIDS Mental Health Project

---

*See also New York City (five boroughs).

Selected Bibliography

THE BOOKS AND ARTICLES listed below are aimed at a broad range of readers, including service providers, researchers, clinicians, and family members. Most discuss family bereavement and grief; others deal with confidentiality, family structure, pediatric AIDS, disclosure, and other psychosocial issues. Sections for children and for parents are included, as well as a videotape listing.

Nonfiction

Balk, D.E., ed. "Special Issue: Death and Adolescent Bereavement." *Journal of Adolescent Research* 6 (1991):1-156.

Bearison, D.J. *"They Never Want to Tell You": Children Talk About Cancer.* Cambridge, MA: Harvard University Press, 1991.

Bergeron, J.P.; Handley, P.R. "Bibliography on AIDS-Related Bereavement and Grief." *Death Studies* 16 (1992):247-67.

Brown, K.H. "Descriptive and Normative Ethics: Class, Context and Confidentiality for Mothers with HIV." *Social Science Medicine* 36 (1993):195-202.

Coles, R. *The Spiritual Life of Children.* Boston: Houghton Mifflin, 1990.

Dane, B.O.; Levine, C., eds. *AIDS and the New Orphans: Coping with Death.* Westport, CT: Auburn House, in press.

Dane, B.O.; Miller, S.O., eds. *AIDS: Intervening with Hidden Grievers.* Westport, CT: Auburn House, 1992.

Demb, J. "Clinical Vignette: Adolescent Survivors of Parents with AIDS." *Family Systems Medicine* 7 (1989):399-43.

Doka, K.J. "Silent Sorrow: Grief and the Loss of Significant Others." *Death Studies* 11 (1987):455-69.

———. *Disenfranchised Grief.* Lexington, MA: Lexington Books, 1990.

———. "Grief Education: Educating About Death for Life." In Anderson, G., ed. *Courage to Care: Responding to the Crisis of Children with AIDS.* Washington, DC: Child Welfare League, 1990.

Dougy Center. *Waving Good-Bye: An Activities Manual for Children.* Portland, OR: The Dougy Center, 1991.

Furman, E. *A Child's Parent Dies.* New Haven, CT: Yale University Press, 1974.

Grosz, J.; Hopkins, K. "Family Circumstances Affecting Caregivers and Brothers and Sisters." In Crocker, A.C.; Cohen, H.J.; Kastner, T.A, eds. *HIV Infection and Developmental Disablities: A Resource for Service Providers.* Baltimore, MD: Paul H. Brookes, 1992.

Levine, C. "AIDS and Changing Concepts of Family." *The Milbank Quarterly* 68 (1990):33-58.

Lipson, M. "What Do You Say to a Child with AIDS?" *Hastings Center Report* 23 (1993):6-12.

Macklin, E. *AIDS and Families.* New York: Harrington Park, 1989.

Michaels, D.; Levine, C. "Estimates of the Number of Motherless Youth Orphaned by AIDS in the United States." *Journal of the American Medical Association* 286 (1992):3456-61.

Nicholas, S.W.; Abrams, E.J. "The 'Silent' Legacy of AIDS: Children Who Survive Their Parents and Siblings," *Journal of the American Medical Association* 268 (1992):3478-79.

Osterweis, M.; Solomon, F.; Green, M., eds. *Bereavement: Reactions, Consequences and Care.* Washington, DC: National Academy Press, 1984.

Pizzo, P.; Wilfert, C.M., eds. *Pediatric AIDS: The Challenge of HIV Infection in Infants, Children, and Adolescents.* Baltimore: Williams & Wilkins, 1991.

Powell-Cope, G.; Brown, M.A. "Going Public as an AIDS Family Caregiver." *Social Science Medicine* 34 (1992):571-80.

Rosen, E. *Families Facing Death.* Lexington, MA: Lexington Books, 1990.

Rosenblatt, P.C.; Walsch, P.R.; Jackson, D.A. *Grief and Mourning in Cross*

Cultural Perspective. New Haven, CT: Human Relations Area Files Press, 1976.

Rosenheim, E.; Reicher, R. "Informing Children about a Parent's Terminal Illness." *Journal of Child Psychology and Psychiatry* 36(1985):995-98.

Siegel, K.; Mesagno, F.; Christ, G. "A Prevention Program for Bereaved Children." *American Journal of Orthopsychiatry* 60 (1990):168-75.

Siegel K.; et al. "Psychosocial Adjustment of Children with a Terminally Ill Parent." *Journal of the American Academy of Child and Adolescent Psychiatry* 31 (1992):327-33.

Walsh, F.; McGoldrick, M. *Living Beyond Loss: Death in the Family.* New York: Norton, 1991.

Simpson, E. *Orphans: Real and Imaginary.* New York: Signet, 1990.

Weller, R.; et al. "Depression in Recently Bereaved Prepubertal Children." *American Journal of Psychiatry* 148 (1991):1536-40.

Wiener, L.; et al. "Pediatrics: The Emerging Psychosocial Challenges of the AIDS Epidemic." *Child and Adolescent Social Work Journal* 9 (1992):381-407.

Fiction

Agee, J. *A Death in the Family.* New York: Putnam, 1955.

Hoffman, A. *At Risk.* New York: G.P. Putnam's Sons, 1988.

Martinac, P. *Home Movies.* Seattle, WA: Seal Press, 1993.

Children's Nonfiction

Bratman, F. *Everything You Need to Know When a Parent Dies.* New York: Rosen Group, 1992.

Draimin, B.H. *Coping When a Parent Has AIDS.* New York: Rosen Group, 1993.

Krementz, J. *How It Feels When a Parent Dies.* New York: Knopf, 1981.

LeShan, E. *Learning to Say Goodbye.* New York: Macmillan, 1976.

Linn, E. *Children Are Not Paper Dolls: A Visit with Bereaved Children.* Incline Village, NV: Publishers Mark, 1982.

Mellonie, B.; Ingpen, R. *Lifetimes: The Beautiful Way to Explain Death to Children.* New York: Bantam, 1983.

Richter, E. *Losing Someone You Love.* New York: Putnam, 1986.

Rofes, E. *The Kids' Book about Death and Dying.* Boston: Little, Brown, 1985.

Children's Fiction

Hickman, M. *Last Week My Brother Anthony Died.* Nashville, TN: Abingdon, 1983.

Viorst, J. *The Tenth Good Thing About Barney.* New York: Atheneum, 1971.

White, E.B. *Charlotte's Web.* New York: Harper and Row, 1952.

Williams, M. *The Velveteen Rabbit.* Garden City, NY: Doubleday, 1971.

Books for Parents

Schaefer, D.; Lyons, C. *How Do We Tell the Children? Helping Children Understand and Cope When Someone Dies* (revised edition). New York: Newmarket, 1988.

Tasker, M. *How Can I Tell You? Secrecy and Disclosure with Children When a Family Member Has AIDS.* Bethesda, MD: Association for the Care of Children's Health, 1992.

Videotapes

Living with Loss: Children and HIV. (Part 4 of the *Hugs InVited* series). Washington, DC: Child Welfare League of America, 1991.

Smith, I. *How Children Grieve.* Portland, OR: The Dougy Center, n.d.

What Do I Tell My Children? Wayland, MA: Aquarius Productions, 1990.

With Loving Arms. Washington, DC: Child Welfare League of America, 1989.

Current Publications

The Changing Role of Volunteerism
Paper Series

This report, based on a conference co-sponsored by the United Hospital Fund, describes the current climate of volunteerism and covers such topics as designing volunteer programs, recruitment and training, and supervising and motivating volunteers. Descriptions are provided of well-managed, creative volunteer programs that have successfully recruited volunteers to meet community needs.

40 pages 1993 $10.00
ISBN: 1-881277-05-4

Friends Like These: A New Breed of Volunteers

The AIDS Friendly Visitor Program at St. Luke's-Roosevelt Hospital Center in New York City is featured in this 15-minute videotape, which describes how volunteers are used to provide needed support to persons with AIDS. Directors of volunteer services and others who work with volunteers should find the videotape useful both as a recruitment tool and as a source of information.

15 minutes 1990 $20.00
ISBN: 0-934459-XX-X

Health Care for Adolescents: Developing Comprehensive Services *Paper Series*

Based on a 1992 conference sponsored by the United Hospital Fund, this paper considers the special health needs of adolescents. Specific problems discussed include AIDS and other sexually transmitted diseases, substance abuse, violence, and mental illness. The paper also addresses the legal and financial barriers to care, describes strategies for outreach and education, and profiles successful service models.

30 pages 1993 $10.00
ISBN: 1-881277-04-6

If We Knew Then What We Know Now: Planning for People with AIDS
Paper Series

This paper grew out of a Fund conference that gathered AIDS service providers and health care leaders from New York and around the nation to discuss what has been learned about designing, organizing, and implementing hospital- and community-based programs for persons with HIV/AIDS.

32 pages 1991 $10.00
ISBN: 0-934459-64-9

In Sickness and in Health: The Mission of Voluntary Health Care Institutions

In this eight-chapter book, leading health care policy scholars and practitioners trace the evolution as well as the sociological, philosophical, and legal basis of voluntary health care institutions. The analyses address the unique mission of these institutions, which are distinguished by their commitment to community service.

256 pages 1988 $35.95
ISBN: 0-07-067532-5

Making Connections: Adult Day Health Care for People with AIDS
A Practical Guide

This manual draws on the experience of model health care programs for people with AIDS. It outlines the philosophy of adult day health care, describes various models, and covers a range of practical issues, including start-up, assessing community need, regulatory issues, staff and space requirements, treatment issues with difficult populations, infection control, and ways to support clients and staff.

40 pages 1993 $10.00
ISBN: 1-881277-14-3

Poverty and Health in New York City

This volume explores the link between economic circumstances and health in New York City and includes chapters on general health status and disability, infant morbidity and mortality, the elderly residing in low-income areas, and avoidable disease and death among disadvantaged groups.

224 pages 1989 $40.00
ISBN: 0-934459-52-5

Simple Acts of Kindness: Volunteering in the Age of AIDS

This book, which discusses the volunteer response to the AIDS epidemic, is based on the proceedings of a Fund conference. In moving first-person narratives, volunteers relate their personal experiences and the rewards and challenges involved in working with a variety of persons with AIDS. Model community- and hospital-based programs that have proved effective in training and involving volunteers are also described.

76 pages 1989 $5.00
ISBN: 0-934459-56-8

The Tuberculosis Revival: Individual Rights and Societal Obligations in a Time of AIDS A Special Report

This report, the product of a distinguished working group, examines the ethical and legal issues that must guide a response to the tuberculosis epidemic. This information is supplemented by case studies and background materials related to the resurgence of tuberculosis in New York City.

64 pages 1992 $10.00
ISBN: 1-881277-12-7

Under the Safety Net: The Health and Social Welfare of the Homeless in the United States

This book draws on the work of 19 programs across the nation devoted to the care of the homeless. Among the topics covered are AIDS; tuberculosis; alcohol and substance abuse; the homeless elderly; mental health; the special needs of women, children, and runaway youth; and the provision of expeditious and economic care. Available from W.W. Norton & Co., 500 Fifth Avenue, New York, NY 10110, or call 1-800-233-4830.

440 pages 1990 $14.95
ISBN: 0-393-30875-8

To order, please write to the Publications Program, United Hospital Fund, 55 Fifth Avenue, New York, New York, NY 10003. Checks should be made payable to the United Hospital Fund and include $3.50 for postage and handling. For information about bulk orders or for a complete list of publications, please call 212 645-2500.

BLACK LABOR, WHITE WEALTH

The Search for Power
and
Economic Justice

Claud Anderson, Ed.D.

PowerNomics Corporation of America
Publisher

OTHER BOOKS AND EDUCATIONAL MATERIALS by Dr. Claud
Published and produced by PowerNomics® Corporation of America, Inc.

Books

Black Reader: Questions You Never Even Thought to Ask **NEW**

PowerNomics®: The National Plan to Empower Black America

Dirty Little Secrets about Black History, Its Heroes and other Troublemakers

More Dirty Little Secrets about Black History, Its Heroes and other Troublemakers

DVDs

Exceptionalism: The Path to Black Empowerment

Vision Beyond the Dream

Inappropriate Behavior: A Roadblock to Empowerment

1866 Indian Treaties: Benefits Due Black Americans

Wake Up America

The Power of Blackness: Reclaiming the Gifts of God

Reparations

On the Firing Line with Questions and Answers

Courses, Videos and other Lectures
www.powernomicstv.com
www.vimeo.com

PowerNomics Corporation of America, Inc. is the *only* authorized publisher and producer of
Dr. Anderson's books and media products.

To find special book and DVD specials and to order, go to www.powernomics.com

a publication of
PowerNomics Corporation of America
<u>Publishers</u>